# Beauty

## A STUDY IN PHILOSOPHY

BY

## Fr. ALOYSIUS ROTHER, S. J.
### Professor of Philosophy in St. Louis University

*IMPRIMI POTEST*

A. J. Burrowes, S. J.
Provincial of the Missouri
Province, S. J.


*NIHIL OBSTAT*

Sti. Ludovici, die 12. Oct. 1916
F. G. Holweck,
Censor Librorum


*IMPRIMATUR*

Sti. Ludovici, die 12. Oct. 1916
✠Joannes J. Glennon,
Archiepiscopus
Sti. Ludovici.

# INTRODUCTION

Beauty is the crowning glory of all things; yet few subjects have been so much misrepresented. Hence the importance and the need of explaining the nature of beauty and of refuting the false theories advanced in regard to it. To do this is the purpose of the following pages.

The study of beauty is, however, beset with peculiar difficulties. For beauty is essentially something spiritual embodied ordinarily in sensible objects. On this account, it readily escapes observation or is confounded with what is sensible. This is why even philosophers have devised so many false theories of the beautiful. But there have been philosophers, such as Aristotle, Cicero, St. Augustine, and St. Thomas, who, by their singular penetration and mature judgment, have eminently qualified themselves to be our masters in the study of this subject. In this treatise we shall follow their example and pass, step by step, from what is evident and on the surface to what is less evident and more scientific. This natural method of procedure will more easily produce conviction and make the

## Introduction

treatise more helpful to the student of philosophy in studying the nature of beauty, and to the student of rhetoric in applying the principles of beauty.

For clearness' sake the leading thoughts will be cast into the form of theses.

# CONTENTS

# BEAUTY

## CHAPTER FIRST

### The Effect of Beauty

**Summary:** Thesis — Proof of thesis — Confirmation of proof.

## THESIS 1

**The beautiful is something which affords delight to the one contemplating it.**

1. **Proof of Thesis.** The truth of this statement appears, in the first place, from a consideration of the *term* beautiful. For the term beautiful is synonymous with the terms delightful, charming, lovely, fascinating, and the like, as every dictionary attests. This shows that according to the common verdict of mankind nothing is regarded as beautiful unless it delights, charms, gives joy. A few illustrations will help to place this inference in a clearer light.

Go out early on a fine summer morning and gaze eastward. A veil of light haze stretches along the line of the horizon; beyond, higher up are scattered about innumerable downy cloudlets forming little groups which look like a flock of lambs grazing in the blue vault of heaven. As you contemplate the spectacle before you the rosy fingered morn begins to touch the haze and the cloudlets, tingeing them with hues and tints so diversified as to fill your whole being with keenest delight and to force from your lips the exclamation, "How entrancing a scene, how beautiful!"

But cast your eyes about you. You are standing beside a lake; its gently sloping shores are overgrown with wild flowers and bushes. Trees here and there stretch their swaying branches over the water's edge. A babbling brooklet runs into the lake not far from you. The air is made vocal by the chirping and the twittering of birds. As the sun rises a fish-hawk is seen poised over the rippling waves and peering into their dark depths below. "It is beautiful," you say under your breath, "it is good for us to be here; how charming, how delightful!"

Now turn to a higher kind of beauty. Yonder stands a cottage; in front of it, under a fruit-laden apple-tree, are seated father and mother in the midst of their rosy-cheeked children. A stranger who happens to pass that way gazes at that peaceful group for a little while and charmed with what he sees utters in a whisper: "How lovely, how beautiful a gathering this is!"

To take one more example from the world of

sound. You are listening to some one whom nature has endowed with a melodious voice. The words he utters charm you even apart from what they convey. The music of his voice fascinates you. Hence you say that he has a beautiful voice.

And why is it that the harmonious maze of many voices or instruments impresses you as beautiful? Is it not because it is "linked sweetness long drawn out"?

So we might go on heaping up instances for ever. We infer thence that the beautiful is always something which affords delight.

2. **Confirmation of Proof.** What each one's personal experience tells him might be confirmed by an appeal to the voice of the past still speaking to us through the signification of the word "beautiful." For the present signification of the word "beautiful" has been handed down to us from the remotest times. Now all the documents, especially those penned by poets, dating back to the very dawn of civilization testify that the term "beautiful" was *only* applied to objects the contemplation of which gratifies, delights, charms, fascinates. And what holds true of the English term "beautiful" likewise holds true of the equivalent terms of other languages, as the Greek καλόν, the Latin "pulchrum," the French "beau," the German "schoen," the Bohemian "krásné," the Polish "piękny," etc.

# CHAPTER SECOND

## Beauty in Relation to the Human Faculties

### ARTICLE 1

#### Beauty in Relation to Sense

**Summary:** Question stated — Thesis — Method of proof outlined — First proof of thesis — Objection to the statement that animals cannot perceive beauty — Objection answered — Second proof of thesis — Third proof of thesis — False views of certain philosophers regarding the relation of sense to the perception of beauty — Beauty often defined in reference to the eye and the ear.

**3. Question Stated.** We have thus established our thesis that the beautiful is something which affords delight to the one contemplating it. The question now arises to which of our faculties the beautiful gives delight. Is it to the cognitive faculties or to the appetitive faculties or to both? But before we can settle this question we must first answer this other, which of our faculties *perceives* the beautiful, the sensitive or

4

the intellectual or both? To this question we
reply:

## THESIS 2

**The beautiful cannot be apprehended
by sense, but by the intellect only.
Hence the delight which the beautiful
affords is not sensible delight.**

**4. Method of Proof Outlined.** Cicero thus
expressed the same idea centuries ago: " Nul-
lum aliud animal (præter hominem) pulchritudinem, venustatem, convenientiam partium
sentit," [1] that is, " No other animal (except man)
perceives beauty, grace, and symmetry of parts."
This passage asserting the inability of animals
to perceive the beautiful supplies the ground for
the proof of the thesis. For if the senses as
such could perceive the beautiful, brute animals
would be able to perceive it too, since they are
possessed of sense organs as well as man. But
how do we prove that brute animals are incapable of perceiving the beautiful? We prove this
from the fact that they never give any evidence
of appreciating the beautiful; for if they give no
evidence of appreciating the beautiful, we are
justified in inferring that they neither do nor
can perceive it.

**5. First Proof of Thesis.** To convince

[1] De Officiis, lib. 1, cap. 4.

yourself that animals never show any signs of appreciating the beautiful, watch them when they chance to be in the presence of things which all regard as beautiful, namely works of art. Did you ever see an animal betray indications of realizing the excellence of a production of art? Did you ever see a brute beast stand awe-struck before a charming picture or statue, or gaze at it in admiration of its beauty? As a matter of fact, if brute beasts are made to look upon a picture, however fascinating, they will show by their utter want of attention and interest that they do not even recognize the resemblance of the picture to any real object. To add a further illustration from the art of music. Grand concerts are often held in parks and other public places; yet no one ever heard of the robins or squirrels or domestic animals streaming thither for the sake of gratifying their esthetic taste. One thing then is certain beyond the shadow of a doubt, that the dumb animals show no indication of appreciating artistic beauty.

But perhaps animals are attracted by the beauty of natural objects. No, neither are they attracted by that. The starry heavens at night are beautiful; the sun sinking below the horizon in the midst of a profusion of flaming clouds is beautiful; the lightning shooting zigzag through the pouring rain is beautiful; yet brute beasts are never seen gazing in mute wonder at these sights, as men often are; if we may judge by external appearances, animals are wholly unaffected by these glories of nature.

We have shown then that brute beasts give no indications of appreciating beauty. From this we further infer that, in point of fact, they do not perceive beauty.— But, you say, this inference is illogical. For granted that animals give no sign of perceiving the beautiful how does it follow that they do not actually perceive it? Might they not be hiding their real emotions?

We reply that such a supposition is preposterous. For it is impossible that the entire animal kingdom should for ages have been filled with delight at the sight of the beautiful, and yet persistently have refrained from expressing this delight outwardly, all the more so as brute beasts have no control over their feelings, but are driven on by irresistible impulse to follow them.

From the fact that animals do not perceive beauty we lastly deduce that they are incapable of doing so. For a natural capacity inherent in an entire class of beings is sure to assert and manifest itself when all the conditions for its exercise obtain, as they certainly do obtain in the case of animals so often placed in the most favorable circumstances for the perception of beauty. It would be an indictment of God's Wisdom to claim that there are in brutes certain instincts or endowments which always have been and still are completely dormant. Consequently our assertion stands that animals and, therefore, the senses cannot perceive beauty. Hence beauty can be perceived by the intellect only, since besides the senses there is no other perceptive faculty in man except the intellectual. It follows further that the pleasure which the beautiful affords *directly* is not sensible pleasure. For the pleasure caused directly by the perception of an object corresponds to the nature of the perception, that is, it is sensible or mental according as the perception is sensible or mental. We say *directly*, for we shall show further on (thes. 7, p. 79) that *indirectly* through the intellect the beautiful, in a way, affords pleasure to the senses.

6. **Objection to Statement that animals cannot Perceive Beauty.** But is it universally true that animals are not attracted by beauty? If they are not attracted by beauty, why do the songsters of our woods warble and trill and pipe in spring and summer so as to turn the orchards and forests and shady groves into veritable temples of song? Again, is it not a matter of common experience that certain animals when they hear harmonious strains of music, as the playing of a lute, stand, as if transfixed, and listen, as if lost in admiration? We are all familiar with the lines of Shakespeare in his " Merchant of Venice " : [1]

[1] Act 5, Scene 1

"For do but note a wild and wanton herd,
  Or race of youthful and unhandled colts,
  Fetching mad bounds, bellowing, and neighing loud,
  Which is the hot condition of their blood;
  If they but hear perchance a trumpet sound,
  Or any air of music touch their ears,
  You shall perceive them make a mutual stand,
  Their savage eyes turn'd to a modest gaze,
  By the sweet power of music."

Further, are there not many animals that love to live in beautiful surroundings? The butterflies and other insects disport themselves amid the most pleasant natural scenery; the humming birds delight to hover on poised wings before the sweet-scented flowers of the honeysuckle; many birds build their nests in the dense foliage of magnificent trees or on the banks of rivers or on the shores of lakes, the very homes of natural beauty. Besides, many animals are of a most graceful form, most tastily adorned with varicolored stripes and spots in divers patterns. Only call to mind the tiger, the leopard, the parrots, the butterflies. Are all these animals insensible to their own beauty and that of their kind?

7. **Objection Answered.** To these apparent objections we reply by granting the facts stated, but by denying the inference thence drawn that brute beasts are capable of appreciating the beautiful. All the indications pointing to a relish of the beautiful on the part of animals are due to

other causes.  But as a satisfactory solution of
this difficulty is important, it will be good to in-
troduce our explanation by something analogous
to the point under discussion. — Suppose you are
in the presence of a man with whom you are not
well acquainted.  You want to find out whether
his senses are in a proper condition.  For that
purpose you hold a little bell before his open eyes;
he shows no sign whatever of seeing the bell.
You conclude from his complete unconcern that
he is blind.  You now sound the little bell; at
once the person's attention is aroused.  Does this
show that you are mistaken and that the man is
not blind?  Not at all; it only proves that his attention was aroused, not by the light from the bell,
but by the sound coming from it.  You vary the
experiment.  You place a piece of paper before
his eyes.  No sign of recognition.  You replace
the piece of paper by a fragrant rose or by a burning coal.  Again the man is all animation.  For
although he cannot see he can smell and feel.
Now apply this analogy to the case under consideration.  Beautiful objects do affect animals,
not, however, just because they are beautiful and
impress the animals as beautiful, but for other
reasons, because those objects excite pleasant sensations in the animals, tickle the palate, gratify
the eye and ear, or prove useful for some purpose
or other, as for food, for shelter, for building
nests, and the like.  Thus birds pour forth their

gladsome notes in order to call their mates or to satisfy an instinctive craving which impels them to fill the air with their song. Or perhaps they are urged on by the Author of nature to sing so charmingly in order to delight man, for whose sake the world has been created. — The playing of a lute causes wanton colts to halt in their wild frolics and listen attentively, because its mellow sweetness soothes their ears. — The butterfly seeks out brilliant flowers to feed upon their nectar or to lay its eggs upon their leaves. — Many animals spend their days in pleasant natural surroundings, because they find there what ministers to their bodily wants. The pleasing and artistic colorings often observable in animals may answer various purposes, as to enable the brute beasts to distinguish one from another more readily, to afford sensible satisfaction to their organs of sight, and no doubt also, to add variety and splendor to the works of nature, in order that man, seeing the beauty of the visible universe, may be filled with wonder and ecstasy and praise the Lord God, the Maker of all things.

We see then that what might seem to be an indication of fondness for natural beauty on the part of animals is traceable to quite different sources.

8. **Second Proof of Thesis.** That animals do not perceive the beautiful can be confirmed by an appeal to common sense or the collective opinion

of men. The argument based on the consensus of men, though not in every case absolutely infallible, nevertheless always carries great weight, as it is very unlikely that so many minds applying themselves to the solution of a question should all be mistaken. — At first sight, it must be confessed, the verdict of common sense would seem to be against us. For if you ask the ordinary man what he thinks beauty is, he will probably answer by giving you some concrete instances of *sensible* beauty. He will tell you perhaps, an ornamented watch is beautiful, or the bright smile of a rosy-cheeked child is beautiful. These answers would appear to indicate that he regards beauty as something sensible and hence perceivable by animals. But no; for if you inquire further whether in his opinion a sheep regards an ornamented watch as pretty or whether he thinks that the pony sees beauty in the smiling countenance of the lad about to leap upon its back, he will think that you are joking. No doubt, people of tidy habits often paint and otherwise decorate places in which animals are kept; they do this, however, not to suit the esthetic taste of the animals shut up in them, but to please themselves and their children and their neighbors. The animals themselves will do their best, as far as lies in them, to destroy every vestige of beauty.— Hence people do not think that animals are capable of perceiving beauty and thus indirectly admit that the beautiful cannot be apprehended by sense as such.

9. **Third Proof of Thesis.** There is still another argument to show conclusively that the senses as such do not perceive beauty. This argument, however, supposes what we shall prove further on in theses 4 and 5. There we shall show that the essence of beauty involves order, proportion, harmony, and symmetry. Consequently, a faculty incapable of apprehending and appreciating these is likewise incapable of apprehending and appreciating beauty. Now order, proportion, harmony, and symmetry are essentially relations, and these sense is unable to perceive. For the senses can, indeed, perceive things which are related, but they cannot perceive relations as such. From this we infer that the senses cannot perceive beauty. Hence our thesis stands confirmed by all those philosophers, as Plato, Aristotle, Cicero, St. Augustine, St. Thomas, and others, who make beauty consist in harmony and proportion. (For quotations from these writers see thesis 4, p. 53 sqq.).

10. **False Views of Certain Philosophers regarding Relation of Sense to Perception of Beauty.** It must be admitted, however, that there are philosophers who regard the beautiful as something appealing solely to our sensuous perception. They are chiefly the sensists and materialists who, as they do not admit any other

knowledge besides sense knowledge, are compelled by the logic of their systems to view the delight caused by the beautiful as a mere sensation. Their mistake in the matter proceeds from a fundamentally wrong system of philosophy which sees no essential difference between sense and intellect; hence their theory must be summarily dismissed.

11. **Beauty often Defined in Reference to the Eye and the Ear.** But if sense is incapable of perceiving beauty, how comes it that the beautiful is not unfrequently defined with reference to the eye and the ear? Thus Webster says: " Beauty is an assemblage of graces and properties pleasing to the eye, the ear, the intellect, the esthetic faculty, or the moral sense." St. Thomas himself gives this definition of the beautiful, " Pulchra sunt quæ visa placent," " Those things are beautiful the *sight* of which pleases." [1] And in another place [2] he tells us: " Isti sensus præcipue respiciunt pulchrum qui sunt maxime cognoscitivi, sc. visus et auditus rationi subservientes," which means, " Those senses chiefly relate to the beautiful which are most highly cognitive, viz. sight and hearing: for they minister to reason " (in the perception of the beautiful).

The answer to this question will be given in another place (thesis 7, p. 79 sqq.), where we

[1] Sum. Theol. 1, q. 5, a. 4, ad 1.
[2] Ibid. 1, 2, q. 27, a. 1, ad 3.

shall speak professedly of the part the senses take in the apprehension of the beautiful. It will suffice here to state that the beautiful is said to be the object of sight and hearing, not because these senses *truly* perceive the beautiful as such, but because they present beautiful objects to the intellect and thus as ministers or instruments of the intellect share, in their own way, in the intellectual delights of the beautiful. Hence it is, too, that St. Thomas in the second passage quoted does not say that sight and hearing *perceive* the beautiful, but merely that they are *related* (respiciunt) to it.

As regards the well-known definition of the beautiful, "Pulchra sunt quæ visa placent," note that the word "visa" in the definition bears a twofold interpretation. First, "visa" may be taken to signify the same as "cognita," the verb "video" often having the meaning of "cognosco." In this acceptation of the particle "visa" the above definition may be rendered thus: "Those things are beautiful the *contemplation* of which pleases." In the second place, we may take "visa" in the literal sense of "seen." Then "pulchra sunt quæ visa placent" should be translated by "Those things are beautiful the *sight* of which gives pleasure" (sc. to the intellect).

It is noteworthy that "sight" alone, and not also "hearing" is mentioned in this definition.

The reason probably is that beauty as perceived by sight is more common and better understood than beauty perceived by hearing. However, beauty of sound is not excluded by the definition; it is merely not expressly mentioned.

## ARTICLE 2

### BEAUTY IN RELATION TO THE INTELLECT AND WILL

Summary: Question stated — Thesis — Preliminary remarks — Ontological truth — Everything is true — Ontological truth in relation to God and creatures — Ontological falsity — The good — Everything is good — Definition and division of love — Wholly unselfish love — Opposite of good, or evil — Opposite of love, or hatred — First proof of first part of thesis — Second proof of same — Third proof of same — No special intellectual faculty needed for the perception of beauty — Proof of second part of thesis — Love of an object not always proportionate to its beauty — How the beautiful contributes to our own good — Two kinds of intellectual delight.

12. **Question Stated.** We have shown thus far that it is the intellect and not sense which apprehends the beautiful, and, consequently, that the delight which the beautiful affords is not sensible delight. The question now awaits solution

to which of the faculties of the soul the beautiful gives delight, whether to the intellect or to the will or to both.   The following thesis states what we think on this question:

## THESIS 3

**The beautiful as beautiful begets intellectual delight only; but in so far as it is identified with the good, it also arouses love in the soul.**

13.   **Preliminary Remarks.**   Before taking up the thesis we must make some general remarks on the *true* and the *good* by reason of the very close connection of these concepts with the beautiful.   In fact so close is the connection that many have identified the beautiful with the true or with the good or with both.

14.   **Ontological   Truth.**   To   understand what is meant by the true we must begin by defining truth in general.   Truth in general is conformity between thought and thing.   This conformity is threefold, namely conformity of thing with thought, called ontological truth; conformity of thought with thing, called logical truth; and conformity of words with thought, called moral truth.   Here we are concerned only with ontological truth or simply the "true."   For, as will soon appear, the truth considered identical with beauty is ontological truth.   Ontological truth

or conformity of thing with a concept (or thought) may be considered under a twofold aspect. For a concept may either serve as a pattern according to which something is made, or it may serve as a norm according to which something is estimated. Thus things are said to be true in the first sense in respect to the Divine concept according to which all existing things have been made, and in general in respect to any concept guiding an artist in his work, as in the examples, " the Universe is true to the concept God has of it," and " the Sistine Madonna is true to the concept of Raphael." — We use truth in the other sense, namely as a norm according to which something is estimated, when we speak v. g. of true friendship, of true humility, of true loyalty. For true friendship, true humility, true loyalty is friendship, humility, loyalty conformable to the concepts of friendship, humility, and loyalty. However, for ontological truth *actual* conformity of a thing to the intellect is not required, it is sufficient that the thing be *capable* of being conformed to the intellect. Hence conformity of thing to thought, whether actual or potential, constitutes the essence of ontological truth. — But ontological truth is also sometimes employed in a less proper sense to designate the object itself which is conformable to the intellect without special regard to its conformity to the intellect. Ontological truth thus taken is rather the matter or foundation on which the relation of ontological truth *strictly so called* is founded; it is what the scholastics call " veritas ontologica fundamentaliter vel materialiter sumpta." This extended use of the term " ontological truth " is, however, very natural and appropriate. For, as we shall explain a little further down, by the very fact that a thing is a thing, it is essentially conformed to the Divine intellect and (to some extent) capable of conforming itself to created mind, therefore ontologically true. Hence " thing " and " the true " are really one and the same, only conceived somewhat differently, " the true " expressing distinctly what " thing " denotes implicitly. Now we can understand how St. Augustine could define the true as " that which is." For he takes ontological truth here for the foundation of ontological truth.

15. **Everything is True.** From the above exposition it readily appears that everything is (ontologically) true. For whatever is, is actually conformed to the Divine intellect and, at least, capable of being conformed to finite intellect. Now since conformity either actual or potential constitutes truth, therefore everything is (ontologically) true. Hence the true is a transcendental notion; for a transcendental notion is one which can be applied to all things whatsoever; and such is the true since, as just explained, everything is ontologically true.

**16. Ontological Truth in Relation to God and Creatures.** It further follows that things are conformed to the Divine intellect necessarily and adequately, for God is infinite; but not so as regards finite intellects, and this for the reason that they are finite. Consequently things are true to the Divine intellect primarily and absolutely, but to created intellect only secondarily and in a restricted sense.

**17. Ontological Falsity.** Now a word about the opposite of ontological truth, namely ontological falsity. Ontological falsity is defined as disagreement of thing with thought. It is clear that there can be no ontological falsity in respect to God, the All-Perfect. As regards finite beings, a distinction must be made according as the thing is referred to the finite intellect as a pattern or as a norm. (See p. 18.) Things referred to finite intellect as a pattern are false when they do not conform to the ideal which the artist has in mind but fails to express. However in this case, common usage does not sanction the word " false," but has settled on other terms. Thus v. g. a picture which falls short of the conception of an artist is not called " false," but a daub, a failure, a bungled piece of work, and the like. But things are called false when not conformed to the intellect as a norm according to which they are judged, as when we speak of a false friend, false virtue, false gods. How-

ever, things are denominated false only meta-
phorically, either because they can prove the occasion of a false judgment or because the mind
has falsely attributed a certain predicate to a certain subject.   For example, a coin is called false
because it is so cunning an imitation of genuine
money as easily to be mistaken for it, and Her-
cules is called a false god because he has been
falsely judged by the pagans of Greece and Rome
to be a god.   The scholastics say that in these
cases things are false " per accidens," not " per
se."   For of themselves (per se) things are
necessarily conformed to the Divine mind and
at least capable, within certain limits, of being
conformed to finite intellect.

18.   **The Good.**   We now pass to the other
concept to be elucidated, namely the good. — The
good in general is that which is suitable to something or perfective of something.   Aristotle de-
scribes it as that which all things crave (id
quod omnia appetunt).   This is an a posteriori
definition of the good, that is, a definition derived
from the effect which the good produces.   For
the good excites a tendency (appetitus), a craving, a longing, a desire, or whatever you may
call it, in the thing for which it is suitable.
Hence it is that desirability (appetibilitas) or attractiveness is regarded as the chief property of
the good.

A thing may either be good in itself (good absolutely) or good to another (good relatively).

19. **Everything is Good.** The statement made by philosophers that everything is good in itself, may sound strange at first, but if rightly understood it is self-evident. For the good has a twofold meaning; it either simply means anything suitable, or it means the same as the perfect. Now it is in the first of these two meanings that we assert everything to be good, not in the second. In other words, we say that everything possesses something that is suited to it, but not that everything is perfect. The statement may be thus rendered more intelligible: In order that a thing may be a thing it must be constituted by something. Now that which constitutes a thing makes it what it is, and what makes a thing what it is, is its essence; and its essence is something suitable to the thing.

Since everything then is good in itself, the good, like the true, is a transcendental concept.

We infer further that since everything possesses some goodness of its own, it can also benefit other beings by communicating its goodness to them. Thus a fly is a source of good at least to its progeny, even though under every other respect it were an utter nuisance. Hence we see that everything is good also in respect to at least *some* other being or beings and consequently relatively good.

20. **Definition and Division of Love.** Since

the good then is that which perfects, it engenders desire and love in rational beings.  We do not consider here in what way non-rational beings are attracted by the good, as the discussion of this question is foreign to our purpose.  And what is love?  Love in general is a certain delight or pleasure the will takes in some good proposed to it, or, as St. Thomas says: " Amor est nihil aliud quam complacentia appetibilis," [1] that is, " Love is nothing else than the pleasure taken in a desirable object."  Love is twofold according to the motive inciting to love.  For we can love an object either for its own sake, for the sake of its inherent goodness, or we can love it because it redounds to our own good, because it is good for us.  The first kind of love is wholly unselfish and hence is rightly called love of *complacency,* which the Standard Dictionary defines as "love delighting in its object for its own intrinsic excellency."  It is also sometimes styled love of benevolence, because it prompts the lover to promote the well-being of the object loved.  The same Dictionary defines love of benevolence as "love seeking to promote the welfare of its object."  If the love of benevolence is mutual it is called love of *friendship.*  For friendship — to quote the Standard Dictionary once more — is "the mutual liking, esteem, or regard cherished by kindred minds as the basis of the mutual in-

[1] Sum. Theol. I, 2, q. 26, a. 1, in corp.

terchange of kind offices." The other kind of love inclining us to seek something as good for ourselves is called love of *desire* or simply desire, yearning, or longing. It may be regarded under a twofold aspect according as its object is licit or otherwise. If its object is licit it is named well-ordered self-love, but if illicit, inordinate self-love. For self-love as such does not necessarily imply anything reprehensible; it is merely "a desire or tending that leads one to seek to promote his own well-being."

21. **Wholly Unselfish Love.** But here a difficulty meets us. We have stated that there is a kind of love which is wholly unselfish. Now is it possible to love anybody or anything with a love that has no admixture of selfishness? Do I not always love another because to love him is beneficial to me? A somewhat fuller exposition of this point is of the greatest importance in this treatise. For we hold that the love of the beautiful is the love of a thing for the sake of its own inherent excellence apart from all selfish consideration. To solve the problem satisfactorily we shall first show that we can love an object for its own sake, on *condition*, however, that the object redounds in some way to our own good. Then we shall answer an objection which might be raised from the apparent incompatibility of the fulfilment of the above condition with *purely* unselfish love.

First, then, we can love an object for its own sake. The voice of mankind vouches for this. For if all love were selfish what would become of the meaning of friendship, which in all languages denotes *disinterested* love between two or more persons? The grandeur of friendship has been exalted to the sky by poets and romancers. Few of their outpourings have met with a readier response than those composed in praise of friendship. Who is there that is not familiar with the old legend of Damon and Pythias, whose heroic fidelity to one another melted the heart of even a tyrant? Recall the magnanimous love of Jonathan for David, the thought of which stirs the soul of everyone who reads the story. "And David and Jonathan made a covenant, for he loved him as his own soul. And Jonathan stripped himself of the coat with which he was clothed and gave it to David, and the rest of his garments, even to his sword and to his bow and to his girdle." [1]— There are other kinds of love besides the love of friendship which, at least generally, are not based on self-interest. There is the love of parents for their offspring. It is not for their own sake that father and mother wish to see their children happy, but for the sake of the children themselves. There is a smile of satisfaction on the lips of the dying father when he sees his son well provided for and successful.

[1] I Kings, xviii. 3 and 4.

The father derives no advantage from the success of his son whom he is about to leave forever; yet he rejoices amid the shadows of death. — Again, every good man loves his fatherland, the country where his cradle was rocked. Is it merely because benefit accrues to him from the country of his birth that he cherishes it? That may sometimes be the case, but by no means always. For in that case, would a man be willing to sacrifice all his goods and lay down his very life for his country, even when its cause seems utterly forlorn and hopeless? — And lastly, are there not many who love their Creator not so much because He is good to them, but because He is so excellent in Himself, so wise, so kind, so mighty, so beautiful?

Moreover, our assertion that we can love others for their own inherent excellence regardless of self, commends itself also on purely a priori grounds. For to be able to love something it is enough that it should, in some way, be good to the lover; it is not necessary, however, that the gain to be derived by the lover from the thing loved be the *motive* or *ground* of his love. It is only when the motive of one's love is one's gain that love is interested.

We have thus shown that it is possible to love another for his own sake. We now pass to the proof of the qualifying clause of the assertion above made, namely that we cannot love another unless such love redounds, in some way, to our own good.

As experience and reason tell us, our will cannot love anything except in so far as it is perfective of us and, consequently, in so far as it is good for us. For if a thing, even though it does us no harm, does not perfect us in any way, it is, as it were, non-existent in regard to us and hence cannot excite our love. It is therefore against the very nature of a rational being to cherish or incline towards something which does not at all perfect it. Hence for an object to be lovable it must be capable of enhancing the excellence of an intellectual being.

But it is objected, if I cannot love an object unless it enhances my own excellence, then, by that very fact, love ceases to be disinterested and becomes interested. We answer that this does not follow. For the aptitude of an object to render a person more excellent *may be*, but is not *necessarily*, the *motive* of the person's love for that object; it may be merely a prerequisite, the ontological ground rendering love possible, a mere condition needed for love to spring up in the heart, and it is only when the perfection of self is the *motive* for loving an object that love is the love of desire or interested love. As long as the perfection of self is merely a condition for loving a thing while the real motive for loving it, is the goodness of the thing in itself,

love is love of complacency or disinterested
love. To illustrate this rather subtle distinction by an example; in order that a piece of
wood may burn, it must be dry; nevertheless
what causes it to burn is not the dryness of the
wood, but the fire to which it has been exposed.
The dryness of the wood merely disposes the
wood for burning. It is a prerequisite, a condition that the wood may take fire. Similarly, in
the case of love of benevolence, what causes a
person to love another is not his own personal
advantage or perfection, but something distinct
from himself, namely the advantage and perfection of another, his own advantage and perfection being merely a condition making love possible. However, it is not necessary that this condition should be explicitly noticed.

What we have just said, has been well sum-
marized by Fr. Palmieri, S. J., in these words:
"Quod bonum ad quod ordinamur sit bonum
nostrum, est conditio quidem cur illud . . . dili-
gamus, non est autem necessario ratio cur dili-
gamus. Ratio enim sufficiens est hæc, nempe
quia est bonum, quæ est ratio formalis volunta-
tis; conditio vero illa, quod nempe sit bonum
quoque nostrum, semper adest, etsi explicite non
consideretur a volente,"[1] which may be rendered
thus: "That the good which nature impels us
to love be our own good, is indeed a condition,

[1] Anthropologia, p. 565.

but not necessarily the reason why . . . we love the good; for, the good being the proper object of the will, the sufficient reason why we love the good is, that it is good. But this condition that the good be also our own good is always present, although it be not expressly adverted to by the person willing." [1]

These abstract statements will perhaps become clearer by showing how the unselfish love of friend for friend, of parent for child, of the patriot for his country, of the virtuous man for God, supposes the good of the lover as a condition.

To begin with the love of friendship. A friend regards his friend as his "alter ego," his other self, in whom he finds his complement and completion. Friends are, so to speak, one soul in two bodies. Hence it is that *true* friendship with the vicious, the depraved, is impossible, since association with such characters, so far from ennobling, is debasing. Mutual perfectibility then is a necessary condition of genuine friendship.

The same holds true in regard to the love of parents. It is a law of nature for parents to cherish *their* children. If they were not *their* children they would not have that peculiar fondness for them which we call parental affection. Parents, in point of fact, look upon their issue as

[1] Cfr. Suarez, De Anima, L. 5, c. 2°; also Lahousse, Psych., p. 442, n. 482.

copies of themselves, as perpetuations of their own personality. This consideration, however, is not the motive of their love, but only a necessary prerequisite for loving their children.

To show that self enters into the love of country we need only recall a few stanzas in which patriots have poured forth their enthusiastic affection for the land of their birth. Listen to Sir Walter Scott's inspired words:

> " Breathes there a man with soul so dead,
> Who never to himself hath said,
> This is *my own*, *my* native land."

Recall the glowing sentiments expressed in our own national anthem:

> " *My* country, 'tis of thee,
> Sweet land of liberty,
> Of thee, I sing."

The lover of his country then considers himself, so to speak, identified with his nation; hence, its progress is his progress; its victories are his victories; its glories are his glories. The patriot's own good is therefore a necessary condition, not the motive, for his ardent attachment to his country.

And finally, as regards the Supreme Being. The love of God for His own sake likewise redounds to the perfection of the lover in innumerable ways. For the God we cherish with such fond affection is *our* God. Do we not pray to Him daily, "*Our Father* who art in heaven"? We are sparks of the Godhead, so to speak. In His infinite perfections, each one of our finite perfections is included in a super-eminent manner. Hence if God is glorified I am glorified; if God is loved I am loved; if God becomes better known I become better known. It is in this manner that when I love God for His own sake, for the sake of His infinite beauty and bounty, I, at the same time, conform to the fundamental law of my nature which prevents me from loving anything except in so far as it is perfective of me. But, to repeat it once more, the longing for my own perfection is not the motive for my loving God, it is merely a condition rendering such love possible.

22. **The Opposite of Good, or Evil.** The opposite of good is evil or bad. Hence evil may be defined as that which is unsuited to something, or that which deprives something of a perfection. Just as a thing can be good in itself or in regard to another, so a thing may be evil in itself or in regard to another. Thus blindness and sin are evil in themselves, a just judge is an evil for a criminal, an energetic school-teacher, for the lazy boy. This shows that what is an evil for another, is often excellent in itself, as the just judge and the energetic teacher in our example.

The definition of evil just given is the definition of evil in the concrete. In the abstract, evil may be described as the privation of a perfection due to a being, i. e. of a perfection which that being ought to have. The absence of a perfection which is not due does not make a thing evil or bad. Otherwise, everything except God would be evil. For every finite being, by the very fact that it is finite, lacks some perfection. Thus man would have to be called evil for this alone that he is devoid of the power of flight, a perfection proper to most birds.

23. **The Opposite of Love, or Hatred.** As the good attracts and begets love, so evil repels and awakens hatred. Hence love and hatred are opposites. It is not necessary to give the various divisions and definitions of hatred, as every one can readily derive them for himself from the divisions and definitions of love by bearing in mind that love and hatred are opposites.

24. **First Proof of First Part of Thesis.** We now return to our thesis in which we state that the beautiful as such has regard to the intellect only.

This can be shown first from the almost universally accepted definition of the beautiful, as the thing the *contemplation* of which gives delight. Hence if we may believe the consensus of men in general, the delight which the beautiful affords is delight springing from contemplation, that is, delight of the intellect.

25. **Second Proof of First Part of Thesis.**

We arrive at the same conclusion by considering what the beautiful is in itself. As we shall show afterwards (thes. 4), the beautiful consists in symmetry, harmony, proportion, order. Now all these constituent principles of the beautiful involve relations and therefore are the objects of intellectual perception only. (Cf. p. 13.) Consequently we are right in inferring that the delight which the beautiful gives is intellectual delight, and intellectual delight only.

26. **Third Proof of First Part of Thesis.** But the strongest proof that beauty appeals to the intellect, and to the intellect only, is drawn from the testimony of consciousness. For, after all, the delight which beauty causes is a phenomenon of our inner self, a manifestation of the soul. Now all manifestations of the soul are taken notice of directly by consciousness, and by consciousness alone. This faculty is therefore the court of final appeal in this matter. We must then carefully look into the inner recesses of our soul and see what goes on there. It is hard at times to arrive at certainty by this process, because the phenomena taking place within our minds are often complicated, fleeting, and transient; none of them is ever seen by itself, but always accompanied, preceded, and followed by others. Hence it often requires an observant and quick mind to fix and hold a psychical phenomenon at all, or, at all events, to fix and hold

it in such a way as not to mix it up with other phenomena connected with it. Our case is similar to that of a person wishing to seize just some one particular fish swimming about in a pond filled with water-lilies, weeds, and the like. He will probably not catch the fish at all, or, if he does, he is likely to take up much other material with it. This is the reason why where consciousness is our only guide, so many mistakes are made in matters of much greater importance than the one under consideration. Hence in order not to be deceived in the search after truth, we must proceed with great circumspection, and in order not to deceive ourselves, we must set about our investigation with candor and singleness of purpose.

Ask yourself then what faculty of your soul feels pleasure when you look, say upon a beautiful lawn. Is it your eye, or is it your intellect, or is it your will? The eye certainly feels pleasure. However, the pleasure it experiences is a mere sensitive pleasure and hence not the pleasure caused by the beautiful. For, as we have shown in thesis 2, the senses as such are incapable of perceiving the beautiful and, consequently, are incapable of enjoying it. Having thus eliminated the senses as *such*, we have narrowed down our discussion to the intellect and the will. We have to make our choice between them, or else admit that both are equally concerned in the enjoyment of the beautiful. It is extremely difficult in this case to make a choice on account of the very intimate connection between the two. For the will follows the intellect; what the intellect pronounces as excellent the will feels prompted to love. Nevertheless if we watch the workings of our soul closely, we find that the delight produced by the perception of the beautiful is not a craving, it is not a tendency, it is not a longing to be united to the object, it is not a rejoicing in the possession of the object, but it is joy arising from merely gazing, an absorption in the sight of the object. Hence the joy is purely intellectual, not volitional; for volitional joy is consequent upon the union of the faculty with its object. I gaze at a foaming waterfall. I do not regard it as perfective of myself; I do not desire it; I do not crave it; I do not tend towards it; I do not want to possess it. I feel delighted in simply looking, gazing. The emotions that begin to stir in the will on beholding the beauty of the waterfall are distinct from the delight of the beautiful. For they are caused, not by the apprehension of the beautiful as such, but by the realization that the beautiful is at the same time good, and the good is the proper object of the will. (Cf. p. 38.)

The conclusion we have arrived at regarding the character of the delight of the beautiful is confirmed by St. Thomas, who, as a sincere and acute analyzer of intellectual phenomena, stands unrivaled. He says: "Pulchrum respicit vim *cognoscitivam;* pulchra enim sunt quæ visa placet,"[1] that is to say, "The beautiful has reference to the cognitive power, for those things are beautiful which please in their very contemplation." And again: "Et sic patet quod pulchrum addit supra bonum quendam ordinem ad vim *cognoscitivam,* ita ut bonum dicatur id quod simpliciter placet appetitui, pulchrum autem dicatur id cujus ipsa apprehensio placet,"[2] which means, "Whence it appears that the beautiful adds to the notion of the good a peculiar relation to the cognitive powers; and while the good is that object which simply gratifies the appetite, the beautiful is that which gratifies by its mere apprehension."[3]

We have thus established our thesis that the beautiful as such appeals to the intellect and not to the will.

27. **No Special Intellectual Faculty Needed for the Perception of Beauty.** The question here suggests itself, Is man possessed of a *special* intellectual faculty for the perception and appreciation of the beautiful distinct from the faculty which apprehends other intellectual objects? There are some who think that man is

[1] Sum. Theol. p. I, q. 5, art. 4, ad 1.
[2] Ibid. p. I, 2, q. 27, art. I, ad 3.
[3] Cf. Rickaby, Gen. Met., pp. 148, 149.

possessed of such a special faculty, which they choose to call "the sense of beauty" or "the sense of the beautiful." Such, however, is not the case. For the beautiful contains none but intellectual elements, namely symmetry, harmony, order. (Cf. theses 4 and 5.) Therefore the intellect is fully competent to perceive these elements and capable of the enjoyment consequent upon that perception. Hence to uphold the existence of such a sense is purely arbitrary; it is to admit a special faculty without any foundation whatever, and according to the scholastic axiom, "Entia non sunt multiplicanda sine necessitate," "Entities should not be multiplied without rhyme or reason." Were we to allow the necessity of a special faculty for the apprehension of the beautiful, why not do the same for the apprehension, say of God, of substance, of accident? Where would we ever stop? However, there seems to be no objection to calling the intellectual faculty as perceptive of the beautiful "sense of beauty," just as the same faculty in so far as it perceives its own proper modifications is called "consciousness." The word "sense" as applied to the intellect thus viewed is by no means inappropriate. For the perception of the beautiful is intuitive knowledge, a sort of intellectual seeing or gazing, and hence bears a great resemblance to sense perception. It is for the same reason that the intuitive power of the mind to perceive certain self-evident truths is called common *sense*.

**28. Proof of the Second Part of Thesis.** We now pass to the second part of the thesis, in which we state that the beautiful, in so far as it is also good, excites love in the will. That the beautiful should excite love in the will is just what we would expect considering the object of the will and the peculiar relation existing between the intellect and the will. The object of the will is the good proposed to the will by the intellect. Hence whenever the intellect apprehends something as good and presents it to the will, the will is attracted by it and drawn to love it. Now the beautiful and the good coincide; for as we shall see in thesis 5, p. 66, the beautiful is the same as the perfect, and the perfect is identical with the good (cf. thesis 3, p. 22). Consequently, as soon as the intellect perceives the beautiful, a tendency arises in the will to love it. The love of the beautiful follows upon the apprehension of it just as the flash does upon the electric spark. Let it be borne in mind, however, that the love we speak of here, is the noblest kind of love of which the soul is capable; it is pure, unselfish love, consisting in the mere volitional gratification of the will, in the mere volitional satisfaction at the superlative goodness of the object contemplated. This sort of love, as will be remembered, is called love of complacency, in contradistinction to the so-called love of desire which regards an object not as good in itself, but as good and useful to the lover. The artist loves the flower in the field because it is so perfect in itself; the gardener loves it because it may prove profitable to him.

29. **Love of an Object not Always Proportionate to its Beauty.** It would seem to follow from what we have just said that the love which a beautiful object enkindles in the will, should be exactly proportional to the intellectual apprehension of the beauty of that object; for beauty arouses love in the will only in so far as it is apprehended. But experience shows that the will does not always love what the intellect apprehends as beautiful. Thus many do not love virtue although they cannot but perceive its excellence.

In regard to this difficulty we say that the love of the beautiful would always precisely correspond to the intellectual perception of it, if the will were at all times under the full control of the intellect and not free, in a great measure, to oppose the attraction of the beautiful object perceived by the intellect. A perverted will, a will which has indulged in unlawful loves, may be at war with its better self and hate what the intellect perceives as beautiful. Nor can the intellect in such a case give itself over unreservedly to its own delights; for the volitional faculty is sure to react on the intellect and hamper it in its enjoyment. The intellectual fruition of the beautiful will thus be marred, since when there is strife in the soul, none of the faculties involved in the strife can receive full satisfaction. In this manner it may happen that, though the intellect sees the beauty of God or of virtue, the will attached to creatures and sense may refuse to be influenced, and may, moreover, like a false friend, bend all its energies to deprive its partner faculty of much of its delight.

30. **How the Beautiful Contributes to our own Good.** We have thus established that the beautiful as beautiful begets intellectual delight only, but that in so far as it is identified with the good it also arouses love in the soul. This love, as we have shown, is love of benevolence and hence entirely unselfish love. Here the question arises how the beautiful contributes to *our own* good; for we pointed out before that we cannot love anything even with the most disinterested love unless it promotes, in some way, our own good. (Cf. thesis 3, p. 26 sqq.) Such a connection between the good loved and our own good, we proved to be a fundamental condition for love to arise in the soul at all.

To this question we reply that the beautiful is in a very marked way our own good, in fact, it is, as it were, part and parcel of our own selves. Hence by loving the beautiful we love ourselves.

To understand this recall the well-known axiom:
"Similis simili gaudet"; "Like loves like."
The truth of this axiom rests on the truth of the
other axiom that every one loves himself. For
what is *like* myself is, in a way, myself, since
there exists, though not a real, yet a logical iden-
tity between myself and what is like myself.
Consequently, by loving what is like me, I love
myself. Now the beautiful is like man's rational
nature, his soul, in a very *special* manner.
Hence by loving the beautiful I love myself.
But how is the beautiful like myself? It is so
because the essence of the beautiful is harmony,
proportion, and order (cf. thesis 4), and the
soul is essentially harmony, proportion, and
order. For the soul is, of its very essence, a
representative principle, i. e. a principle which
through its faculties exhibits a likeness or simili-
tude of things. In this sense the soul might be
rightly called a *harmony*, to use an expression
employed by the Pythagoreans, though in a somewhat different sense. Moreover, the intellect is
essentially a reasoning faculty. Now reasoning
is a complex, yet at the same time, a most *orderly*
process. For it consists in comparing two ideas
with a third and then drawing a conclusion according to the principles: " Two things identical with a third are identical with each other,"
and " If one of two things is identical with a
third thing and the other is not, then those two

things are not identical with each other." Hence the soul, on account of this its orderliness and harmony, is like the beautiful objects which it perceives, and therefore it is that the will loves the beautiful so exceedingly. The orderliness and harmony of the soul then is a condition, a prerequisite for the soul to love things beautiful.

What we have just said may be confirmed by a sentence of Fr. Liberatore S. J.[1] He says: " Quod si causam quæris cur de claritate et proportione facultas cognoscitiva oblectetur, ea non incongrue esse dicitur, quia in tali objecto cognoscitiva facultas aliquid sibi simile reperit; similitudo enim causa est amoris et complacentiæ," that is to say, " If you ask the reason why the cognitive faculty takes delight in clearness and proportion, it would seem to be that the cognitive faculty finds in such an object some likeness to itself; for likeness is the cause of love and satisfaction."

31. Two Kinds of Intellectual Delight. Here we must draw attention to a source of possible confusion. We said that the delight of the beautiful is intellectual delight. But, some one might ask, is there not intellectual delight which does not spring from the contemplation of beauty? Thus the solution of a difficult mathematical problem is often accompanied by intense intellectual delight; yet this delight is evi-

[1] Met. Gen. c. 1, a. 8, n. 54.

dently not the effect of the perception of beauty. Is there any way of discriminating between this kind of intellectual delight and the intellectual delight produced by the contemplation of beauty?

As regards this point we say that there are two kinds of intellectual delight. The one kind springs from the mere discovery of the truth (v. g. of a complicated mathematical problem), and implies reasoning. It might be called the delight of "pure knowledge." The other kind of intellectual delight arises from the apprehension of what is symmetrical, harmonious, proportionate, in a word, of what is beautiful, and as such does not imply reasoning. For the perception of the beautiful is mere contemplation or intuition, mere viewing or gazing. To mark the difference between this kind of mental delight and that springing from the mere discovery of the truth, the word "contemplation" has been introduced into the definition of the beautiful; for the beautiful is defined as that the *contemplation* of which affords delight. Nor is it difficult to point out some of the characteristics distinguishing the delights of the intellect upon the discovery of the truth, from the delights of the intellect upon the apprehension of the beautiful. The delights which accompany the discovery of the truth are keen and stirring, the delights which attend the apprehension of the beautiful are gentle and soothing. The pleasures of pure knowledge may be experienced by the most perverse, the hard, the cold, the cruel; they may be felt by the penetrating intellect of the tyrant when he has hit upon some ingenious plan of ridding himself of a rival. But the satisfaction proceeding from the sight of the beautiful is the portion of the imaginative, of the generous, of the affectionate. Mere knowledge, deep and penetrating, may lead to hatred; the perception of beauty gives birth to love. Thus we see that there is a notable difference between the delights of knowledge and the delights caused by the sight of beauty. The delights attending the contemplation of beauty might not be ineptly called the joy of the mind, the jubilation of the intellect.

However, before leaving this question, a word of explanation is needed. We stated above that the delight accompanying the solution of a difficult mathematical problem is not the delight peculiar to the beautiful. When we say this, we do not mean to assert that there is no beauty in mathematics or in science in general. Far be it from us. All we mean to say is that the pleasure accompanying the mere investigation and apprehension of truth is a pleasure of its own, distinct from the pleasure proper to the perception of the beautiful. But the scientist does not merely investigate and apprehend the truth; he does much more. He arranges and combines the truths apprehended into systems according to some rational principle, and thus erects ideal structures truly beautiful, structures the contemplation of which fills him and all his fellow scientists with exquisite delight. The very expressions used to describe science — as, knowledge reduced to law, knowledge coordinated, arranged and systematized — indicate that order, the essential element of beauty is a distinctive feature of science (cf. thesis 4, p. 52 sq.). It was the recognition of the beauty in science which made Ben Jonson consider poesy as the soul of science when he wrote:

"O sacred poesy, thou spirit of Roman art,
The soul of science, and the queen of souls."

The pleasure of scientists in the prosecution of truth and their delight in the contemplation of a scientific system may be compared to the pleasure the builders of the cathedrals of the Middle Ages felt in the work of construction and the delight they experienced in gazing upon the finished structures.

# CHAPTER THIRD

## The Essence of Beauty in General

### ARTICLE I

#### Order Essential to Beauty

**Summary:** Question stated — Thesis — Divisions of beauty — Definition and divisions of order — Precise meaning of thesis determined — A posteriori proof of thesis — Confirmation of proof — A priori proof of thesis — Thesis corroborated by authority — Exceptions to thesis merely apparent.

**32. Question Stated.** Thus far we have spoken of beauty in its relation to the faculties which it affects. In the next two theses we shall consider beauty as it is in itself, in its inner nature and essence.

## THESIS 4

### Beauty essentially implies order.

**33. Divisions of Beauty.** Before proceeding to the proof of the thesis we must set down the chief divisions of beauty, as we shall have frequent occasion to refer to them in what follows.

46

In the first place, beauty is either *uncreated* or *created*. The former is peculiar to the Deity, the latter belongs to His handiwork, creatures.

Another division of beauty is into *spiritual* and *material* beauty. Spiritual beauty is the beauty of spiritual entities, whilst material beauty is the beauty of corporeal things.

Spiritual beauty, in turn, is either *intellectual* or *moral*, according as it regards intellectual or moral excellence. A genius, for instance, possesses intellectual beauty, a magnanimous man, moral beauty.

Beauty is also divided according to the nature of the beautiful object into *supersensible* and *sensible* beauty. If the beautiful object lies beyond the perceptive power of sense, as God, beauty is supersensible, if it lies within the sphere of sense, as a violet, beauty is sensible.

Sensible beauty is sometimes subdivided into beauty of *color* and beauty of *sound*, and into beauty of *form* and beauty of *movement*. The beauty of mathematical construction falls under the beauty of form.

A further division of beauty is into *ideal* and *real*. Ideal beauty is peculiar to creations of the mind, to things in so far as they are objects of thought, as the ideals in the mind of God or the conceptions of an architect guiding him in the exercise of his art. Real beauty, on the other hand, is the beauty of things regarded in themselves. This may be subdivided into *natural* and *artistic* beauty, or the beauty of the works of nature and the beauty of works of art.

The last division of beauty is that into *symbolic* and *intrinsic* (non-symbolic) beauty. A thing possesses symbolic beauty in so far as it is the symbol or emblem of an object which is beautiful in itself; but when the object is beautiful in itself, and, as it were, in its own right, and not precisely as suggesting something else, it is said to possess intrinsic beauty. One and the same object may possess both these kinds of beauty. Thus a lily is beautiful in itself and also as the emblem or symbol of the beautiful virtue of purity.

**34. Definition and Divisions of Order.** Prior to entering upon the proof of the thesis, it is further necessary to explain the notion of order.

Order is defined as the arrangement of several things according to some common principle. For order then we must have several things. One thing, it is plain, cannot be set in order. Supposing I have but one dot (A) on a piece of paper, order in regard to this dot is inconceivable. But even if I have several things and these things are placed at random, no one will say that they are arranged in an orderly way. Hence that there may be order, several things must be disposed according to some relation or common principle. Suppose v. g. that to the dot (A) two more dots (B and C) be added at equal distances from (A), then these three dots form an orderly arrangement. Because several things are now arranged according to a given relation, namely equality of distance. — Take another more complex example. As everybody will admit, there is order in a watch. And why? Because, in the first place, there are many parts in a watch, as the wheels, springs, levers; and because, in the second place, these parts are all arranged and combined for a common purpose, namely to cause the hands of the watch to move in such a way as to indicate the correct time. Order then is the unification of the manifold, multiplicity reduced to unity.

Having thus explained the notion of order in general, we shall now give a few of the divisions of order.

Order is either *simple* or *compound*. Order is simple when things are ordered according to one principle only, and it is compound when ordered according to more than one principle. Thus if I arrange the books in a library according to their subject only, the order is simple; but if I arrange them according to their subject, language, and size, the order becomes compound. The order of the universe is most complex, God, the great Orderer disposing and unifying the endless multiplicity and variety of things in a most marvelous manner.

A further division of order is into *statical* and *dynamical* order. Statical order obtains among things that are fixed, as the orderly arrangement of a Byzantine cathedral, while dynamical order attaches to things in motion, as the movements in a dance or the evolutions of an army drawn up for drill.

Again, order is *necessary*, when it arises from the essences of things, as the moral order; and *changeable* (contingent), when founded on some non-essential principle.

Another very important division of order is that into *symmetrical* and *harmonious* order. Symmetrical order results from the regular repetition of equal or similar parts, but in opposite directions. Thus the orderly arrangement of the parts of the human body is symmetrical, because one side of the body is the exact counterpart of the other. Harmonious order arises from the balancing of dissimilar elements in such a way as to produce an agreeable impression. The seven colors of the rainbow and the combination of sounds in a good musical performance are instances of harmonious order.

Lastly, there is a species of order in which the principle of order is some end to be obtained. An example of this kind of order is the order which a general establishes when drawing up his troops for battle, or the order which a good ruler maintains among his subjects for the securing of their temporal happiness. The gaining of the victory and the procuring of the temporal happiness of the governed, are the ends determining the arrangement of the general and the regulations of the governor respectively.

35. **Precise Meaning of Thesis Determined.** We are now ready to establish the thesis in which we stated that beauty essentially implies order. All we mean to maintain in this thesis is that where there is no order there can be no beauty. Note that there may be no order in an object for two reasons, either because there is merely and simply an absence of order in the object, or because there is actual disorder in it. In the first case, the expression "no order" is taken negatively, in the second, positively. Our contention is that lack of order either negative or positive is incompatible with beauty, but with this difference, that where there is a mere absence of order, an object is simply *un*beautiful without being ugly, whereas when there is disorder, the object is positively ugly.

36. **A Posteriori Proof of Thesis.** Our first argument shall be drawn from experience. Consider a single point on a sheet of paper out of all relation to any other point. No one will call this point beautiful; nor is it ugly; it is simply

unbeautiful. Were you to add other points so
as to form a perfect circle, there would be order
and beauty. — Or suppose some one were to direct your attention to a single stone in a stately
building and then ask you, "Is that stone beautiful?" you would answer, "Not in itself, but
as a part of the whole structure." — To add one
more example: A single sound in a symphony
considered apart from all the other sounds is
not thought by any one to possess beauty. — Observe, however, that what is simple and devoid of
order under one aspect, may be complex and arranged in an orderly way under other aspects
and so far forth beautiful. All we mean to say
here is that a thing, *in so far* as it is out of all
relation to other things, is not deemed beautiful.
It is hardly necessary to prove that, where there
is positive disorder, there is not only no beauty,
but actual ugliness and unsightliness. This will
be best brought home by an instance or two. —
Take the statue of a man with the eyes of unequal size, bulging out, and very far apart from
one another. Every one will pronounce the face
of this statue ugly. — And what is it that makes
poor music so offensive to the esthetic sense? Is
it not want of harmony, want of a proper combination of notes?

37. **Confirmation of Proof.** Some addi-
tional light may be thrown on our assertion that
beauty implies order, by a consideration of the

tendency of the human mind to discover order in things. — Consciousness tells us that the mind delights in discovering unity amid variety, in unifying the manifold. This discovery of unity amid variety, this unification of the manifold is one of the chief charms of scientific pursuits. Now unity amid variety constitutes order. Since then the natural propensity of our minds leads us to ferret out the hidden order of things, it would seem to follow that unless an object exhibits an orderly arrangement of parts, we can take no pleasure in contemplating it, in other words, we can see no beauty in it.

**38. A Priori Proof of Thesis.** It can also be shown a priori that there can be no beauty without order. — The human mind is an intellectual faculty; hence it estimates things according to their proper worth. Now a thing which is in a state of disorder or confusion is positively defective. How then can the intellect be charmed by it? Again, since order is one of the chief excellencies of things, is it surprising that the mind should be left cold and indifferent in gazing upon a thing that is so simple, so plain, so uniform, as not even to possess the first element of order, namely a multiplicity of parts?

**39. Thesis Corroborated by Authority.** Lastly, it will be well to confirm our arguments from reason by an appeal to authority. Many of the most distinguished philosophers of both ancient and modern times tell us that beauty essentially implies order, or, what comes to the same thing, proportion, symmetry, fitness, unity in variety, and the like. It is not, however, our intention to indorse the views of all these philosophers in *every* respect. We quote their words merely to show that, to their minds, beauty essentially implies order.

Let us begin with Plato. According to Plato the essence of the beautiful lies in the fitness and symmetry resulting from the relation of the concept to the plurality of phenomena.[1] Aristotle, Plato's disciple, tells us: " The chief elements of beauty are order, symmetry, and definiteness "[2]; and again: " Beauty implies a certain magnitude and order."[3] Cicero shall be our next witness. He says: " Sicut corporis est quædam apta figura membrorum cum coloris quadam suavitate, sic in animo opinionum judiciorumque æqualitas et constantia cum firmitate quadam et stabilitate virtutem subsequens aut virtutis vim ipsam continens, pulchritudo vocatur,"[4] which may be rendered thus: " Just as in respect to the body, a certain apt configuration of the members together with a certain charm of coloring is called beauty, so also in regard to the soul, the equipoise and harmony of views and

---

[1] See Ueberweg, History of Philosophy, v. 1, p. 129.
[2] Met. 3, 1078, n. 361.
[3] Poet. chap. 7.
[4] Tuscul. quaest. 4, c. 13.

judgments either springing from virtue or constituting the very essence of virtue is called beauty." St. Augustine, who was a great philosopher as well as a great theologian, has the following: " Quid est corporis pulchritudo? Congruentia partium cum quadam coloris suavitate." [1] In English, "What is bodily beauty? The harmonious arrangement of parts with a certain charm of coloring." In another place [2] he defines beauty in general as the " splendor ordinis," "the splendor of order," a definition so pithy that it has become famous. St. Thomas asserts in a number of places that beauty consists in order, proportion, and the like. Thus in his Sum. Theol. he states: " Unde pulchrum in debita proportione consistit [3]; " Hence beauty consists in proper proportion." In another place of the same Sum. Theol. we read: " Ad pulchritudinem tria requiruntur, primo quædam integritas sive perfectio . . . et debita proportio sive consonantia et item claritas " [4]; that is: " For beauty three things are required, first, a certain integrity or perfection, . . . secondly, due proportion or harmony, and lastly clearness." From among the modern philosophers we single out Fr. Tongiorgi S. J., who has obtained a wide and well-deserved rep-

[1] Epis. 3, n. 4.
[2] De. Ver. Relig. c. 4, n. 77.
[3] Sum. Theol., p. 1, q. 5, ad 1.
[4] Ibid., p. 1, q. 39, a. 8.

utation for his philosophical acumen. He says:
" Pulchritudinis essentiam atque intima constitu-
tiva continet celebris ex Platone et Augustino
definitio, ' unitas in multitudine et varietate,' qua
nulla verior et pulchrior excogitari potest," [1]
which is translated: " The essence and inner-
most elements of beauty are contained in the
famous definition of Plato and Augustine, ' unity
in multiplicity and variety,' than which no truer
and more beautiful definition can be thought
out." We shall conclude the list of authorities
by three quotations from well-known writers on
the Beautiful in the English language. S. T.
Coleridge, quoted in Webster's Dictionary says:
" The old definition of beauty in the Roman
school was ' multiplicity in unity,' and there is
no doubt that such is the principle of beauty."
The " Vocabulary of Philosophy " under
" Beauty " states that " according to Hutchison
the general foundation and occasion of the idea
of beauty is uniformity and variety." Words-
worth speaks of the " production of beauty by a
multiplicity of symmetric parts, uniting in a con-
sistent whole." [2]

**40. Exceptions to Thesis merely Apparent.**
But here a serious doubt interrupts our progress:
though it is true that order or unity amid variety
is often discernible in beautiful objects, yet there

[1] Ontologia, n. 307.
[2] Cf. Webster's Dictionary under " Beauty."

seem to be many exceptions to the rule, and if so, order cannot be considered essential to beauty, since nothing can be without that which is essential to it.  It will be convenient to set down a few of these apparent exceptions and test them.

The full moon is certainly beautiful; poets have sung of its charm since time immemorial, and yet, so our objector says, the full moon presents itself to the beholder as a mere flat, almost undiversified, luminous disk hanging in the sky. Where is there sufficient variety here for order? Hence order would not seem to be necessarily required for the beautiful.[1]

This objection rests on a misconception.  For we must not consider the moon by itself, but together with its surroundings.  Look at the moon on a bright, cloudless night.  Behold the circular disk as it sends forth its soft light and moves slowly through the mighty dome of heaven, while on the earth below everything is bathed in its mellow rays.  Or watch it when the sky is partially overcast; see how it sails through the clouds, now half-hidden, now disappearing altogether, now reappearing again. — In this view, the moon certainly presents enough variety to render it exceedingly beautiful.

A green lawn, not variegated with flowers, is deemed beautiful, and yet — so some think — there is no variety here.

[1] See Urráburu, Ont. p. 533.

As regards this instance, we wish to note first that we must not confound the pleasure of the beautiful with the agreeable sensation certain colors produce in us. Just as sugar is pleasant to the taste, so certain colors are agreeable to the eye. But this sensible pleasure does not constitute the pleasure of the beautiful, as some have imagined. (Cf. p. 120.) However, we think that a green lawn is not only agreeable to the sight, it is likewise truly beautiful. For it shows forth unity amid variety. It is formed of many blades, each symmetrical in form, broader at the base and tapering to a point. The upper side of each leaflet is of a different shade of green from the lower. Perhaps a gentle breeze is stirring the grass causing it to sway to and fro in graceful movements. Moreover — and this is very important in the present case — by reason of the pleasant sensation produced by the sight of the lawn, the mind is enabled to perceive that green is adapted or suited to the eye, and adaptation or suitability always implies order. (Cf. thesis 7, part 2.) It is not true, then, that a green lawn is beautiful without presenting the necessary elements of order. It must not be supposed, however, that the intellect always adverts to the elements of order in an object explicitly and by a reflex act; no, as a rule it takes them in intuitively, very rapidly, and almost unconsciously; that is sufficient for the appreciation and enjoyment of the beauty of an object. — We shall add one more instance from the region of sound. One single tone can be beautiful. Here again, there would seem to be beauty without variety. In answering this difficulty, we might repeat (mutatis mutandis) what we said in respect to a single color (green), namely that we must not confound the agreeable with the beautiful, and that the perfect adaptation of a single sound to the ear is alone sufficient to impart beauty to the sound. (Cf. thesis 7, p. 74.) But a single tone taken in its isolation can also be called beautiful, because, even considered in itself, it exhibits order or unity amid variety. For in every note we can discern at least three elements, namely pitch, intensity, and timbre. Now these elements may be blended and correlated according to certain proportions, and a good ear detecting these proportions will discern beauty in a single tone. Moreover, on hearing a sweet, musical note, the musician may recall pleasing airs heard before, and thus the single note becomes beautiful by association. (See thesis 8.) Hence the aforesaid exceptions to the general statement that beauty essentially implies order, are exceptions only in appearance.

## ARTICLE 2

### BEAUTY THE SPLENDOR OF ORDER

**Summary:** Transition to new phase of subject — Thesis — Meaning of thesis illustrated — A posteriori proof of thesis — A priori proof of thesis — Answer to query — Authorities vouching for truth of thesis — Corollary: Scale of beauty — Relationship between the true, the beautiful, and the good.

**41. Transition to New Phase of Subject.** We have thus established the thesis that there can be no beauty without order. We next ask: Is any kind of order sufficient to constitute beauty? To this question we answer:

### THESIS 5

Beauty as such consists not in any kind of order but in order that is resplendent, or, to use an expression of St Augustine, in the "splendor of order."

**42. Meaning of Thesis Illustrated.** Our contention then is that it is only order of a certain degree of perfection which constitutes the beautiful. Nor should this seem strange; for there are many things which consist in a quality of a certain degree of intensity. Thus genius is *exalted* intellectual power, *remarkable* aptitude for some special pursuit; patriotism is *devotion* to one's country, i. e. *ardent* love or affection for one's native land.

43. **A Posteriori Proof of Thesis.** Our first and strongest argument is based on experience. Make two points (A and B) upon a piece of paper. There is order here; for the one point may be regarded as standing in relation to the other according to a certain principle, v. g. it may be regarded as just above or below the other, or so many inches to the left or the right of the other; yet no one perceives any beauty in the simple arrangement. Join the two points by a straight line. There is order in a straight line as the very name " straight " indicates. Still we think we will not be contradicted if we say that a *mere* straight line is not regarded as beautiful by people generally. Now add a third point (C) at equal distances from the other two (A and B) and draw two straight lines from C to A and B. The resulting figure will be an isosceles or equilateral triangle. Now order becomes more pronounced and beauty begins to appear. Continue to render the figure more complex by turning one of the lines, say AB, about the point A, and now look at the diagram thus obtained; it is a perfect circle; all its parts are disposed in a definite order about a point called the centre; it looks beautiful.

The more complex and well-made a mathematical construction, the more it charms, provided, of course, that the relations of the parts to each other and to the whole are clearly perceived by the beholder. So much beauty is there in mathematical figures that the type of beauty according to many is a wavy line called the "line of beauty." We see now that order of a certain degree of complexity is required for beauty. Hence it is, too, that things which are plain and unadorned, as a plain house, a homely dress, a simple knife, are regarded as possessing beauty either in no degree or, at best, in a very low degree.

**44. A Priori Proof of Thesis.** The thesis may also be established a priori from the consideration of the definition of beauty thus: Beauty is defined as that the contemplation of which affords *delight* to the intellect. Now delight is not an ordinary, weak affection of the soul, it is an affection of a certain intensity. But an intense emotion requires a proportionate cause. Hence it stands to reason that only order of some degree of perfection can give rise to the pleasure of the beautiful.

**45. Answer to Query.** But here a difficulty arises: if beauty is order of *some degree* of perfection, how can I ever know whether an object possesses the degree of perfection required to make it beautiful? and if I cannot know that, how can I know whether an object is beautiful or not?

To this inquiry we reply: It is, indeed, hard at times to point out the exact line of demarcation between what is beautiful and what is not beautiful, but it by no means follows that we can never distinguish the beautiful from the non-beautiful, as will readily appear from a few parallel instances. Who can tell just when dawn ends and day begins? Can we therefore never discern dawn from day? The colors of the rainbow shade very gradually one into the other, and yet no one will deny that there is a certain number of distinct colors in the rainbow. The boy becomes a youth and the youth a man; but can any one indicate the exact second or minute when this takes place? There may be doubt at times whether a certain object is beautiful or not, when it lies in the region of transition from non-beauty to beauty; but in *most* instances persons of some discernment can readily tell whether an object gives intellectual delight or not. They will tell you that a Corinthian column is beautiful while a plain pillar used for support is not, that a mansion built in Queen Anne's style is handsome, while a square brick house is not, and so forth and so forth.

**46. Authorities Vouching for Truth of Thesis.** Nor is our thesis without the support of eminent authorities. We have already quoted

the words of St. Augustine in the formulation of
the thesis. According to Plato, beauty is the
"*splendor* veri,"[1] " the *splendor* of (ontological)
truth." This definition is less explicit than that
of St. Augustine, but it amounts to the same
thing. St. Thomas has the following: " Ratio
pulchri in universali consistit in *resplendentia*
formæ super partes materiæ proportionatas et
super diversas vires et actiones," that is to say:
" The general character of the beautiful is the
*splendor* of the form in different parts of matter
or in different powers and activities."[2] In another place St. Thomas cites the pseudo-Dio-
nysius in favor of this view. He says: " Ad
rationem pulchri duo concurrunt secundum Di-
onysium, sc. consonantia et claritas."[3] This
means, " The essence of beauty requires two
things, namely proportion and lustre." According to Leibnitz beauty is the perfection of things
which, inasmuch as it is apprehended, affects us
with pleasure.[4] We shall conclude with a quo-
tation from Fr. Rickaby, S. J., which, besides giving his own view, also contains the opinions of
two other English authorities in regard to the
point at issue. He says: " There must be an

---

[1] This definition of beauty, though not found in any
of Plato's works, has been ascribed to him by tradition.
It is certainly the definition of the Platonists. (See
Urráburu, Ont. p. 529.)

[2] Opus, " De Pulchro et Bono."

[3] Sum. Theol. p. 1, q. 39, a. 81.

[4] Cf. Am. Cath. Quart. 1885, p. 724.

element of *distinction,* as Mr. Arnold would have said, of *lustre,* as Mr. Faber puts it ; and this . . . *distinction,* or *lustre* is often supplied by some pleasing instance of 'unity in variety,' which many make to be the very definition of the beautiful." [1]

**47. Corollary: Scale of Beauty.** It follows as a corollary from the thesis that the greater the perfection of a thing, the greater is its beauty. As there is an ascending scale of perfection in creation, so is there of beauty. Beauty is lowest in the mineral kingdom, higher in the vegetative and animal kingdoms, and highest of all in men and angels ; while above all these, as the source of all beauty, is the infinite beauty of the Creator Himself.

**48. Relationship between the True, the Beautiful, and the Good.** This would seem to be the proper place to point out more explicitly the relationship which exists between the true, the beautiful, and the good. Are these three concepts and their objects the same or are they different ?

In the first place, the *concepts* of the true, the beautiful, and the good are certainly not the same. For if they were the same, it would be inexplicable why there are three distinct terms in every language corresponding to the English "the true, the beautiful, the good," as "verum,

[1] Gen. Met. p. 151.

pulchrum, bonum " in Latin, " τὸ ἀληθές, τὸ καλόν, τὸ ἀγαθόν " in Greek; " le vrai, le beau, le bon," in French; " das Wahre, das Schoene, das Gute," in German, etc. etc. — The same also appears from the consideration of the ordinary meanings of these three terms. For a thing is called a true thing, in so far as it is conformable to the idea of itself; it is called beautiful, in so far as its contemplation affords delight to the beholder, and it is called good, in so far as it is suited to something and excites desire. — But if we regard the true, the beautiful, and the good in themselves, then the true and the good in one of their significations are identical with the beautiful, and in another they differ from it. For the true sometimes denotes the same as that which is conformable to the Divine ideal, and hence denotes the same as the perfect; and the good sometimes signifies the same as that which possesses whatever it should have, and hence likewise signifies the same as the perfect. (Cf. thesis 3, p. 17 sqq.) The true and the good taken in these two meanings respectively are identical with the beautiful or perfect. But frequently the true means anything that is knowable, even though it be very imperfect, and the good anything that possesses reality, even though it is devoid of some perfections it should have. Thus understood, the true and the good are, of course, not identical with the beautiful. For the beautiful

is always something perfect in its kind.  From
the above it is also seen that one and the same
thing may at once possess truth, beauty, and
goodness, but under different aspects.  For example, a spirited race horse is a true horse, because it is conformable to the idea of a horse ; it
is beautiful, because it is a perfect horse, and it
is good, because it is desirable to its owner.  It
is on account of this close relationship of these
concepts that Plato couples τὸ καλόν and τὸ ἀγαθόν,
and that Goethe and Cousin class together the
true, the beautiful, and the good.

# CHAPTER FOUR

## Prerequisite for the Enjoyment of Beauty

**Summary:** Thesis — Thesis explained — Obstacles to proper appreciation of beauty — Sense in which beauty may be called relative.

## THESIS 6

**Beauty, in order to be fully appreciated and enjoyed, must be clearly perceived by the mind.**

49. **Thesis Explained.** This statement, although self-evident, may be thus brought into clearer light. In order that beauty may be appreciated and enjoyed it must be presented to the mind. Now it is presented to the mind by knowledge. Hence the more clearly the beautiful is known, the more it will be appreciated and enjoyed. The clear perception of beauty is therefore a necessary requisite or condition for relishing beauty.

50. **Obstacles to Proper Appreciation of Beauty.** But there are many obstacles both on the part of the object and on the part of the mind

68

on account of which the beautiful often remains hidden from the beholder. One of the principal obstacles on the part of the object is the very excellence of the beautiful. The arrangement of the parts of an object, although most orderly in itself and most perfectly adapted to the end for which the object is intended, is at times so complex, so intricate as to baffle the penetration of the observer. Here is an ingeniously constructed machine. It is really beautiful, but the ordinary man sees no beauty in it, because he fails to understand its workings. Certain games, as baseball and football, seem meaningless and devoid of beauty to the uninitiated, yet to him who understands the purpose of the distribution of the players, their shrewd tactics, and dexterous movements, such sports possess a great charm. But it is chiefly beauty in nature that is often of such excellence as to remain unrecognized. The more we search into the works of nature, the more beauty they reveal to our gaze. And no wonder; for they are the handiwork of the infinite Artist whose designs and purposes no finite mind can fathom.

The beautiful is furthermore not always duly appreciated, because it is not properly manifested through the medium of speech and the other signs which serve as vehicles for the expression of beauty. Thus a poem, or statue, or painting, no matter how exquisite in its external finish, affords but little esthetic delight if it expresses the artist's idea or ideas obscurely and vaguely.

Lastly, a want of proper appreciation of the beautiful is often traceable to the partial or total absence of taste. Taste is defined as " the faculty of the mind by which we both perceive and enjoy whatever is beautiful, harmonious, and true in the works of nature and art, the perception of these qualities being attended with emotions of pleasure." (See Standard Dictionary.) Taste for beauty, though found in most men in some measure, is very rarely found in a high degree of perfection. That such should be the case, is in full accord with the ordinary dealings of Divine Providence which bestows with a less lavish hand gifts intended chiefly for the enjoyment of men, such as wit, a talent for music or poetry, and also a taste for beauty.

51. **Sense in which Beauty may be Called Relative.** What has just been said shows beauty to be something relative in the sense, that the appreciation and enjoyment of beauty is greater or less according to the greater or less capacity of the agent for such appreciation and enjoyment.

# CHAPTER FIVE

## SPECIAL KINDS OF BEAUTY

### ARTICLE 1

#### SENSIBLE BEAUTY

**Summary:** Preliminary remarks — Thesis — Precise meaning of sensible beauty — Proof of first part of thesis — Proof of second part of thesis — The two aspects of sensible beauty illustrated — Several difficulties answered — First scholium: Light and sensible beauty — Second scholium: How the senses can be said to enjoy the beautiful — Higher and lower senses in relation to sensible beauty — Sensible beauty and touch — Dangers incident to contemplation of sensible beauty.

**52. Preliminary Remarks.** After developing the elements of beauty in general, we shall next take up the consideration of a particular kind of beauty, namely sensible beauty, which, on account of its special connection with us men, calls for separate treatment. If sensible beauty is true beauty it must, of course, embody all the essential elements of beauty, and this it does, as we shall show in the next thesis.

## THESIS 7

Sensible beauty is of two kinds, the
one *absolute*, found in the sensible
object considered in itself, the other
*relative*, found in the sensible object
in its relation to sense. Absolute
sensible beauty consists in regularity
of form, in the symmetrical arrangement of colors, and the harmonious
combination of sounds; relative sensible beauty consists in the due adaptation of the sensible object to the
organs of sense.

53. **Precise Meaning of Sensible Beauty.**
Note first that, when we speak of sensible beauty,
we do not mean beauty perceived by sense, but
beauty perceived by the intellect in the objects
of sense. For we showed before (thesis 2) that
the senses as such are incapable of perceiving
beauty.

54. **Proof of First Part of Thesis.** The
thesis has two parts. In the first part we state
that there is beauty in the sensible objects themselves and that this beauty consists in regularity
of form, the symmetrical arrangement of colors,
and the harmonious combination of sounds.
That there is beauty in the sensible objects themselves needs no proof, as it is admitted by all ex-

cept those who erroneously maintain that beauty is not objective. (See thesis 12.) That there is a kind of sensible beauty which consists in regularity of form, symmetrical arrangement of colors, and the harmonious combination of sounds, is shown by experience. Take a sensible object which is universally regarded as beautiful, one of those butterflies which everybody instinctively pronounces beautiful, pretty, handsome, for example the swallowtail or the painted beauty, so common both in North America and in Europe. What is it that pleases us so much in these butterflies? It is their regularity of form and the symmetrical arrangement of their coloring. The two halves of these winged creatures are perfectly alike, the fore wings and the hind wings on the right being perfect counterparts of the fore wings and the hind wings on the left. Further, there are all sorts of markings on the wings and the bodies, as bars, bands, eyes, spots of diverse colors often shading insensibly one into another all arranged in most consummate harmony.

The beauty of a sensible object is greatly enhanced by the graceful movements of its parts. A beautiful object constantly changing in form without losing its symmetry and harmony is, as it were, equivalent to a number of beautiful objects presenting themselves in succession to the eye. Look at a pair of leopards disporting themselves

in their cage; how much their gambols and antics
add to the beauty of their bodies. This is also
the charm of certain drills, as of a corps of cadets
or of a squadron of cavalry. The beauty of such
drills is chiefly due to the multiplicity of symmetrical groupings incessantly varying.

As regards sound, the same holds true. A
beautiful musical composition is characterized by
the exact proportion in which the various sounds,
often consisting of a veritable maze, stand to one
another. Good music essentially implies concord
and harmony.

**55. Proof of Second Part of Thesis.** We
now come to the second part of our thesis where
we state that there is another kind of sensible
beauty, which belongs to the object regarded in
its relation to sense and consists in the adaptation
of the sensible object to the organ of sense.
Adaptation of one thing to another, the accurate
adjustment of means to an end, especially where
this adjustment is of a somewhat intricate character, is always indicative of purpose and orderly
arrangement, and hence always impresses us as
beautiful. There is beauty in the ingenious
mechanism of clocks and other skilful contriv-
ances, because they answer their purpose so well.
—The eye, so wonderfully fitted for the end intended by the Creator, is very beautiful indeed.
If it does not strike us as such, the reason is that
we do not sufficiently understand the marvelous

suitability of this organ for its functions. Now
objects of sense are likewise suited or adapted to
our senses, and that often in a singular manner.
A fresh rose gratifies the eye and the smell; the
nightingale's song soothes the ear. But the rose
and the nightingale's song could not produce these
pleasant effects if they were not *adapted* to the
sense of sight, smell, and hearing respectively.
The mind perceiving this adaptation or suitability
or adjustment finds it beautiful. Note, we do not
say that the pleasure which the senses experience
constitutes beauty; for beauty is not sensible
pleasure; but this pleasure is a token of the adaptation of the object of sense to the organ of sense,
and it is this adaptation which the mind considers
as beautiful. Nor does beauty become merely
subjective on this account, since it is not the subjective pleasure which we regard as beautiful, but
the (objective) adjustment of the object to the
organ; the pleasure merely reveals the existence
of the adjustment. Now we can readily see why
even a single color or a single note should affect
us as beautiful, as the uniform tint of a single
petal or a single sound of the human voice. We
now understand, too, why attractiveness or charm
of coloring, and sweetness or agreeableness of
sound enter as elements into several definitions of
corporeal beauty given by eminent authorities.
Thus Cicero in the 4th Tusculine disputation defines this particular kind of beauty as " the apt

configuration of the members together with a certain charm (suavitas) of coloring." (See p. 54.) St. Augustine [1] asks the question, " What is bodily beauty? " and he answers, " The harmonious arrangement of parts with a certain charm (suavitas) of coloring." (See p. 55.)

**56. The Two Aspects of Sensible Beauty Illustrated.** Of these two phases or aspects of sensible beauty, the absolute and the relative, sometimes the one and sometimes the other predominates, whilst sometimes they are equally or nearly equally blended. Take a Gothic cathedral with its arches, buttresses, and windows all symmetrically disposed, and with its turrets, steeples, and spires soaring towards the sky. It is beautiful in very deed, but its beauty is chiefly architectural, resulting from the graceful and artistic arrangement of its parts. In like manner, the charm of a concert is principally due to the intricate maze of sounds combined in perfect unison. On the other hand, the beauty of a smooth lawn, of the blue vault of the sky, of the individual notes of a flute or an organ is mainly traceable to the perfect adaptation of certain colors and sounds to the eye and ear respectively. Objects symmetrical in arrangement and suited to sense, in about an equal degree are, for instance, a garden well laid out or a piece played on a sweet violin by a skilled performer.

[1] Epist. 3, 4.

**57. Several Difficulties Answered.** The twofold aspect of sensible beauty will explain away a difficulty which might be urged against the view that makes beauty consist in order. For some one might say, Are there not many objects which are symmetrical in form and yet are regarded as ugly, as a toad, the face of the monkey, certain kinds of insects, and the like? Thus Shakespeare in " As You Like It," [1] says:

> " Sweet are the uses of adversity
> Which like the toad *ugly* and venomous
> Wears yet a precious jewel in her head."

Ennius [2] calls the monkey " a very *ugly* beast " (turpissima bestia).

To meet this objection we must first distinguish between intellectual beauty and sensible beauty. The animals mentioned are all very beautiful from the purely intellectual standpoint. Their structure, like that of any other of God's creatures, is most wonderfully adapted to the end of their existence, as every scientist will readily admit. But they do not possess sensible beauty. This is partly due to the fact that they affect the sense of sight disagreeably, just as certain gaudy colors do. Hence these objects are not adapted to our sense of sight. The intellect, discovering this want of adjustment by the unpleasant sensation their aspect produces, pronounces them ugly, so far as their *sensible appearance* goes.

[1] Act. 2, Scene 1.
[2] Ann. 11, 15.

The Author of nature has established this disproportion between sense and object in certain cases for wise reasons of His own, often unknown to us. One of the reasons for His doing so is perhaps, to enhance the beauty of beautiful sensible objects by contrast. We admit, however, that the aversion we feel for certain things is often traceable to other causes, as ignorance, prejudice, custom, fear, and the like. We attribute to certain objects disagreeable or hurtful qualities, and then, viewing them in the light of our subjective conceptions, regard them as ugly. But these causes alone do not explain why we turn from certain things at first sight with an instinctive disgust and loathing, of which with the best of intentions we cannot rid ourselves.

**58. First Scholium: Light and Sensible Beauty.** To complete our thesis we must add a few remarks. — First of all, we wish to direct attention to the part which light plays in the domain of sensible beauty. It not only reveals the grace of form and the delicacy of coloring, but it itself, if not too intense, delights the eye. Only think of the mellow glow of dawn, of the glory of the setting sun, or of a landscape sleeping in the sunlight. Nor should we forget the share which shadows have in enhancing the sensible beauty of objects. How beautiful a grove looks late in the afternoon with all its trees painted in shadows upon the grass as if by an invisible hand.

59. **Second Scholium: How the Senses can be Said to Enjoy the Beautiful.** Another remark we wish to make here regards the question whether and to what extent the senses can be said to enjoy the beautiful. It is plain that the senses cannot enjoy the beautiful *of themselves;* for, as we have shown in thesis 2, the senses as such cannot apprehend beauty; hence neither can they relish it. But this does not show that the senses are unable to enjoy the beautiful in so far as they administer to the intellect. For by ministering to the intellect they become, so to speak, united to it, one with it, and in virtue of this union are elevated to a higher plane. Thus they become capable of doing what of themselves they could not do, just as matter which of itself is incapable of feeling, becomes capable of it by its substantial union with the soul.[1] This would seem to be the reason why so many definitions of beauty state expressly that the beautiful gives delight to the eye or to the ear, as the definition of St. Thomas, " Pulchra sunt quæ visa placent," " Those things are beautiful the *sight* of which affords delight "; and the definition of Webster quoted before, " Beauty is an assemblage of graces and properties pleasing to the *eye,* the *ear,* the intellect, the esthetic faculty, or the moral sense." In fact St. Thomas tells us in as many words that the senses take de-

[1] See Liboratore, Psych. n. 72.

light in what is proportionate and hence beautiful. For he says: "Unde pulchrum in debita
proportione consistit, quia sensus delectantur in
rebus debite proportionatis . . . ,"[1] that is to say,
"Hence the beautiful consists in due proportion,
because the senses are delighted at things which
are proportionate . . ."

That sight and hearing can enjoy the beautiful
as instruments of the intellect can also be shown
in a slightly different way thus: There can be
no doubt, in general, that the mind can influence
the body. The blush of modesty or of shame,
the pallor of fear, the trembling of the limbs at
the thought of danger, bear witness to this. Why
then should not something similar happen in our
case? Why should not the intellectual perception of beauty react on the eye and the ear and
produce in them delights which are not their
own, but which are communicated to them by the
intellect? The eye and the ear present beautiful
objects to the intellect; and the intellect, in its
turn, floods these senses with pleasures of singular delicacy and refinement.

What we have said of sight and hearing applies also, and even more, to the imagination and
fancy. For the imagination is, as it were, the
storehouse of all the other senses. It preserves
the impressions made on the other senses and
reproduces them either spontaneously or at the

[1] Sum. Theol. p. 1, q. 5, art. 4, ad 1.

beck of the will.[1]   Further, it is not only capable
of reproducing former sense impressions; it can
likewise recombine, in new and original ways,
the elements furnished by the senses, slough off
what is commonplace, jarring, ugly in them, and
transform, exalt, and glorify the outer world entering into it through the portals of the outer
senses.  The creative power of the imagination
is the birthright of the poet who fashions for
himself and his readers a world even more beautiful than the real, everyday world in which we
live.  The fancy differs from the imagination
chiefly in this that it is more playful, airier, less
deep, less serious than the imagination.

60. **Higher and Lower Senses in Relation
to Sensible Beauty.**  But what is the reason
that, when treating of the enjoyment of the beautiful on the part of the senses, we only refer to
the higher senses of sight and hearing and not
also to the three lower senses of smell, taste, and
touch?  The reason for this is that the lower
senses, although they relish the beautiful, do so
much less perfectly than the higher senses.  The
great superiority of the higher senses over the
lower in the enjoyment of beauty appears from
the unequal capacity of the different senses to
perceive proportion or order.  True, none of the
senses can apprehend order as such and in the
abstract — that is the exclusive prerogative of

[1] Cf. Lahousse, Psych. n. 102.

the intellect. Nevertheless the eye, the ear, and the imagination can apprehend order in the concrete, and that to a very high degree. No doubt, a relation of parts is often perceived by means of the lower senses, but of so vague and confused a character as hardly to deserve the name of beautiful. Moreover, the subjective element in the case of these senses often predominates to such an extent as to divert the attention almost entirely from the object and the diversity of its parts and qualities. When a man eats a luscious pear, what he adverts to chiefly is the taste, the object itself is hardly noticed. We admit, however, that by each of the lower senses the mind can apprehend a sensible object as suited to the organ of sense and so far forth as beautiful. Still custom does not sanction the application of the word beautiful to objects of the lower senses, not because they are devoid of all beauty whatever, but because they possess only that special kind of sensible beauty which consists in the adaptation of the object to sense. We call perfumes *agreeable,* viands *delicious,* a cooling breeze *refreshing,* rather than *beautiful.*

What we have just said accords fully with what St. Thomas tells us: " Ad rationem pulchri pertinet quod in ejus aspectu seu cognitione quietetur apprehensio; unde et illi sensus *præcipue* respiciunt pulchrum qui maxime cognoscitivi sunt, sc. visus et auditus rationi deservientes; dicimus enim pulchra visibilia et pulchros sonos. In sensibilibus aliorum sensuum non utimur *nomine* pulchritudinis. Non enim dicimus pulchros sapores et odores,"[1] which may be rendered thus: " When we speak of the beautiful we mean something the sight or perception of which quiets the apprehensive faculty. Hence those senses *chiefly* regard the beautiful which possess cognitive capacity of the highest degree, namely sight and hearing as ministering to the intellect. For we say that sights are beautiful and that sounds are beautiful. But in respect to the sensible qualities perceived by the other senses, we do not make use of the *word* beautiful; for we do not say that tastes and odors are beautiful." Note in regard to this passage — St. Thomas does not say that the eye and the ear *only* relate to the beautiful, but that they do so *chiefly* (præcipue), nor does he say that tastes and odors are not beautiful, but that we do not use the *word* beautiful in regard to them.

61. **Sensible Beauty and Touch.** To avoid confusion we must add some explanation in regard to the sense of touch. This sense perceives objects as soft, smooth, cooling, warm, light, and the like, but it also perceives them as extended, as possessing parts outside of parts. Now when we say that objects of touch are not called beautiful, we mean to say that the word beautiful is

[1] Sum. Theol. 1, 2, q. 27, art. 1, ad 3.

not applied to them in so far as they are soft, smooth, cooling, warm, light, or possessed of similar qualities. But they may be truly called beautiful when presented to us by the sense of touch as being made up of parts. For in so far as touch perceives parts outside of parts, it can perceive proportion in the concrete just as the eye can, and hence offer to the intellect an object truly beautiful. Thus a blind person, by passing his hand over a well constructed, raised mathematical figure, can trace the relations of the parts of the figure to each other and in this manner apprehend it as beautiful.

**62. Dangers Incident to Contemplation of Sensible Beauty.** This seems to be an appropriate occasion for making a few remarks on the dangers of contemplating sensible beauty, especially human sensible beauty. It is well for us to know whence these dangers arise, lest what is the crowning glory of a thing should prove a pitfall and a curse. The reason for the slipperiness of sensible beauty is not far to seek. The perception of sensible beauty is always accompanied by sensible gratification of the eye and ear or imagination. Now sensible gratification, even when lawful, is liable to suggest and pave the way for gratification that is unlawful and thus often leads the unwary into deplorable excesses. Hence Jeremias cries out: "Death is come up through our windows "[1] i. e. through our eyes. This, it seems to us, explains why so many poets have an unsavory reputation in morality and why so much poetry, both ancient and modern, is sensual and unreadable. This only proves the truth of the ancient maxim: " Corruptio optimi pessima," " The best thing, when not used in the right way, becomes the most loathsome." It further shows that the Author of nature who made things beautiful for wise reasons of his own, nevertheless wishes us to use much caution and moderation and good sense in viewing sensible beauty. However, what we have said of the contemplation of sensible beauty does not at all apply to the consideration of beauty in general and of spiritual beauty. On the contrary, the thought of the beauty of God, of virtue, of heroism, has a most refining, elevating, and exalting influence. Hence it is that some of the most upright of men, as St. Thomas and St. Augustine, have written most forcibly and eloquently on the subject of beauty.

[1] Jerem. ix. 21.

## ARTICLE 2

### SYMBOLIC BEAUTY

**Summary:** Importance of consideration of symbolic beauty — Thesis — Elucidation of thesis — Symbolic beauty a particular case of association of ideas.

**63. Importance of Consideration of Symbolic Beauty.** Besides sensible beauty, sensible objects also possess symbolic beauty. As this kind of beauty renders sensible objects suitable for the expression of the highest kind of beauty, namely spiritual beauty, it will be well to treat of it in a special thesis.

### THESIS 8

**Sensible objects, besides their own inherent beauty, also possess symbolic beauty.**

**64. Elucidation of Thesis.** A symbol is "anything that (not being a portrait) stands for something else and serves either to represent it or bring to mind one or more of its qualities."[1] Hence symbolic beauty is the power an object has of suggesting or bringing to mind beauty which lies outside and beyond itself. To establish our

[1] Standard Dictionary.

thesis then we must make it clear that sensible things can signify or express beauty which is not their own. That they can do this can be easily shown. For, in the first place, sensible objects often bear a natural relation, as of coexistence, cause or effect, to some beautiful object. Look at yonder bridge sweeping in graceful curves from pier to pier over the broad expanse of the Mississippi River. The bridge is beautiful in itself, but it likewise speaks to you of the genius of its architect, and of the energy, industry, and civilization of the people who promoted the erection of the imposing structure. It thus opens out a vista of beauty lying beyond its stone piers and steel spans and trusses and trestles and the seething and gurgling waters beneath. Or watch that buoyant life-boat shooting swiftly and securely along the rocky coast of the ocean. It is a thing of beauty; it looks like a gull cutting through the foaming waves. But this life-boat can tell a story that conjures up pictures of still greater beauty — of how in a stormy night it cleaved its way through the surging, pounding billows and carried off a precious burden of many lives from a foundering ship. Or gaze up at the castle there built on a jutting rock centuries ago. How its lofty keep, its many towers round and square, its parapets and battlements, all symmetrically arranged, delight the eye! But it also recalls the days of yore, the days of the minstrels, of the troubadours, of the minnesingers; it reminds you of tilts and tournaments fought within its walls and of many a gallant deed in championship of defenseless innocence and knightly honor.

The above are instances in which the connection between the sensible object and the beauty symbolized is natural. Often, however, this connection is conventional or, at best, rests on some remote and fancied resemblance; nevertheless the beauty symbolized is frequently of a most supersensible and exalted nature. Thus the lily is regarded as the symbol of purity; the rose, of love; the violet, of modesty; the lamb, of meekness; the lion, of courage; the oak, of strength. A piece of silk ornamented with stars and stripes has been chosen by the United States to represent her might, her majesty, her honor, and whatever else is dearest to her. All the above symbols have each a sensible beauty of their own, but the sensible beauty inherent in them is greatly enhanced by their suggestion of spiritual beauty.

Symbolic beauty is sometimes possessed even by things which do not themselves appeal to the senses. For even an unsightly object may suggest something very beautiful. Here is a gray-haired old man lying stretched out in his coffin. The pale, emaciated countenance is not beautiful; but it reminds you of a career well-spent, of devotion to duty, of fortitude in adversity, of moderation in success; it speaks to you with an eloquent tongue of the beauty of a good and noble life. — The carnage after a battle is horrid to behold; it brings tears to the eyes, it sickens the heart; yet it has its beauty. For it manifests to you the love of country that burned in the breasts of these heroes now lying stiff in death before you.— Isaias tells us of the Man of Sorrows during the hours of his passion: "There is no beauty in him nor comeliness, and we have seen him and there was no sightliness that we should be desirous of him." [1] And yet that same Man of Sorrows was never more beautiful than in those dread hours. For his bruises and wounds said to all who could understand: "Greater love than this no man hath than that a man lay down his life for his friends." [2]

65. **Symbolic Beauty a Particular Case of Association of Ideas.** It will be well to note here that the connection in virtue of which sensible beauty suggests invisible beauty is but a particular case of association of ideas, by which is meant "any connection or relation between objects or ideas that unites them in thought."

[1] Isaias liii. 2.
[2] John xv. 13.

## ARTICLE 3

### BEAUTY PROPER TO MAN

**Summary:** Transition to new subject — Thesis — Proof of thesis from consideration of fine arts — A priori proof of thesis — Thesis as a corollary — Synonyms of beauty — The sublime — The opposite of the beautiful, or the ugly.

**66. Transition to New Subject.** We have seen that sensible beauty can be and often is symbolical. There now arises a question of prime importance to us as men. Is there among the various kinds of beauty one which is peculiar to human beings, one which is, as it were, their birthright and appeals to them in a special manner? We shall give our answer to this query in our next thesis.

## THESIS 9

**The beauty which gives the highest satisfaction to *man* is spiritual beauty expressed by means of an appropriate sensible symbol.**

**67. Proof of Thesis from Consideration of Fine Arts.** We shall show the correctness of our thesis, first, by a consideration of the fine arts, since they are acknowledged by all to be the very embodiment of the beauty which appeals most to man. Let us start with music. Take a composition by one of the great masters. Why does it give such exquisite delight? Because, by means of melodious and harmonious sounds, it expresses some exalting or inspiring idea, such as love, hope, kindness, pity, mercy, and the like, and through this idea stirs the heart to emotion. Good music then is a sensible symbol of a supersensible conception. Music which does not express an idea is mere pleasing sound, mere empty jingling possessed of but little beauty. That the function of genuine music is really such as just described, may be confirmed by its definition as " the science combining tones in melodious, rhythmic, and harmonious order so as to excite the emotion and appeal to the intellect." [1]

What holds true of music holds true likewise of painting, a graphic art, and of sculpture, a plastic art. The finest paintings and sculptures are those which fitly symbolize some spiritual conception. Take the Sistine Madonna regarded by everybody as one of the most beautiful paintings ever produced by the genius of man. The painting derives its charm chiefly from expressing on canvas the stainless purity of the Virgin and her tender maternal love for her Infant Son. So true is it that the beauty of painting and sculpture

[1] Cf. Americ. Encyclop.

is the symbolization of spiritual conceptions, that some of the most valuable pictures and statues are mere personifications of abstract qualities or ideas, such as faith, hope, charity, liberty, courage, etc.

As regards architecture, another of the fine arts, almost the same remarks will apply. A cathedral looming up before you, symmetrical, well-proportioned, harmonious, majestic, is beautiful to behold. But its visible beauty becomes transformed into the beauty of a higher order, when you have grasped the meaning of the stately pile before you, when you come to consider it as the emblem of the invisible, of something lying beyond the ken of the eye. " This is no other than the house of God and the gate of heaven." [1] All the excellence and magnificence of a cathedral is but a tribute to the Great Architect of the universe. The massive walls tell of God's power, the broad dome, of His immensity, the lofty roof and towers, of His majesty, the multifarious decorations, of His lovableness. This is the full significance of the architectural beauty of a temple of the true God.

Finally, we must add a word more about poetry, which is universally regarded as the special realm of the beautiful. What is poetry? It may be defined as " the form of literature that embodies beautiful thought, feeling, or action in

[1] Gen. xxviii. 17.

melodious, rhythmical, and (usually) metrical language, in imaginative and artistic construction" (Standard Dictionary). The secret of poetry then consists in presenting to the mind of the reader some beautiful conception by the aid of language. Now language, while essentially a sensible symbol of thought, is at the same time a symbol so flexible, so pliant, so adaptable, as to lend itself to the expression of every thought and of every shade and nicety of meaning. A good poet turns all the advantage to be derived from a skilful handling of speech chiefly to a twofold use.

First by means of speech he calls up in the imagination and fancy sensible scenes which themselves are emblems of beautiful ideas. The whole sensible universe lies open before the poet; he now carries you up to the starry heaven, now he takes you down into the caverns of the earth, now he conducts you into the open fields and the darkling woods, now he makes you navigate the stormy seas; and all this in order to lead you into regions of spiritual beauty. — Similar to this device of the poet for conjuring up visions of beauty, is the use of figures of speech, such as metaphor, metonomy, synecdoche, the chief charm of which consists in associating the immaterial with the material.

In the second place, the poet presses into service all the aids which language, regarded as mere material utterance, offers for the better and more effectual expression of thought. Hence he builds up his sentences most artistically, he marshals his words into verses which please by their rhythm, he chooses words and assemblages of words which are music to the ear. Who can point out all the artifices of the poetic genius to set aflame the imagination of the reader and to communicate to him his own conceptions, ardor, and enthusiasm?

We see then that the delight of poetry results from the expression of beautiful thoughts through the apt use of symbolism.

**68. A Priori Proof of Thesis.** The argument just given in proof of our thesis is an a posteriori argument. We can also prove our contention a priori thus: The human mind in its present state of union with the body cannot exercise its functions unless aided by sense cognition. Such is the dependence of man's intellectual activity on sense conditions, that even when engaged in most abstract speculations, the mind cannot dispense with the services of the imagination. No doubt, this dependence is only extrinsic, but it is true dependence nevertheless. Hence it is that thinking fatigues the brain and that when the imagination is deranged, thought cannot go on properly. No wonder then that the spiritual must be clothed in appropriate sensible symbols before the intellect can realize and enjoy it. For in this way abstract beauty is, as it were, rendered concrete and thus brought down to the level of man and placed within his reach. Disembodied spirits are not hampered by such restrictions, but man, the lowest of intelligent beings, cannot soar into the regions of beauty without the aid of his lower nature.

**69. Thesis as a Corollary.** Lastly, our thesis follows as a corollary from a previous consideration. For, as stated (p. 79 sq.), the delight which the intellect derives from the contemplation of the beautiful, in a manner, overflows and pours itself out into the sensitive and material part of our compound nature. Now such a communication between the immaterial and material part in man could hardly take place unless there were some intervening bond to bridge over the chasm between intellect and sense, and this bond is the sensible symbol under which beauty presents itself. It is by means of this bond that it becomes possible for sense life to share in the pleasures of the intellect.

**70. Synonyms of Beauty.** Before leaving this thesis dealing with the nature and kinds of beauty, it will be useful to direct attention to some of the synonyms of the adjective beautiful, namely, beauteous, handsome, pretty, fair, lovely, comely, graceful, and picturesque. But first observe that beautiful itself is used in two meanings. Sometimes beautiful merely expresses in the concrete what beauty taken in its greatest generality expresses in the abstract. In this meaning the word beautiful is not synonymous with the aforenamed adjectives, but denotes the genus under which the concepts signified by those adjectives fall as species or varieties. It is thus that the term beautiful has been employed hitherto. But frequently it has a specific meaning, just as the term animal besides its generic meaning of sentient being has also the specific meaning of *irrational* sentient being. Beautiful in this specific sense signifies "possessing the noblest and most spiritual beauty which affords the highest satisfaction to the mind." Now it is in this signification that beautiful is synonymous with the eight terms just enumerated. As there is question here of the common meaning of words we shall let a dictionary, the Century, speak for us: "*Beauteous* is chiefly poetic and covers the less spiritual part of the beautiful. *Handsome* is founded upon the notion of proportion, symmetry, as the result of cultivation or work. A handsome figure is strictly one that has been developed by attention to physical laws into the right proportions. It is less spiritual than beautiful. A handsome face is not necessarily a beautiful face. Handsome applies to larger and more important things than pretty, as a handsome house; a pretty cottage. It is opposed to homely. *Pretty* applies to that which has symmetry and delicacy, a diminutive beauty without the higher qualities of gracefulness, dignity, feeling, purpose, etc. A thing not small of its kind may be called pretty if it is of little dignity or consesequence; as a pretty dress or shade of color; but it is not used of men or their belongings, except in contempt. *Fair* starts from the notion of brightness that catches the eye; it notes that sort of beauty which delights the eye by complexion and feature. In this sense it is now less common in prose. *Lovely* is a strong word for that which is immediately pleasing to the eye; it applies primarily to that which excites admiration and love. *Comely* applies rather to the human figure, chiefly to its proportions; it is used less commonly than handsome to express the result of care and training. *Graceful* is used particularly of motions, looks, speech, as a graceful walk, a graceful deportment, a graceful speaker, a graceful air. *Picturesque* is applied to objects forming or fitted to form an interesting or striking picture, as a mountain, a water-fall, a pine-covered headland, a gay costume amid appropriate surroundings."

71. **The Sublime.** There still remains another concept closely allied to the beautiful which claims our attention, namely the *sublime*. The sublime may be defined to be that which is so perfect as to surpass the comprehension of the one

contemplating it.[1] For this reason the sublime strikes the mind with a sense of grandeur and power, physical or moral, and awakens sentiments of awe, veneration, and the like. Comparing the concept of the sublime with that of the beautiful we find that they at once agree and differ: they agree in this that they both relate to perfection; and they differ in this that the perfection which the sublime regards passes beyond the ken of the human mind and can only be partially apprehended by it, whereas the perfection which constitutes the beautiful lies wholly within the reach of man's comprehension and can be easily and clearly grasped and understood. Hence it is that the effects produced in us by the contemplation of the sublime and of the beautiful are quite unlike. These different effects of the sublime and the beautiful have been excellently set forth by Hamilton. He says: " The feeling of pleasure in the sublime is essentially different from our feeling of pleasure in the beautiful. The beautiful awakens the mind to a soothing contemplation; the sublime rouses it to strong emotion. The beautiful attracts without repelling, whereas the sublime at once does both; the beautiful affords us a feeling of unmingled pleasure, in the full and unimpeded activity of our cognitive powers; whereas our feeling of sublimity is a mingled one of pleasure and pain,

[1] See Urráburu, Ont. p. 546.

—of pleasure, in the consciousness of strong energy, of pain, in the consciousness that this energy is vain." [1]

72. **The Opposite of the Beautiful, or the Ugly.** Before concluding this thesis it will be well to add a few remarks on the opposite of the beautiful, namely the ugly, the unsightly or deformed; for a concept is often rendered clearer by contrasting it with its opposite. — Since the beautiful is agreeable in appearance and pleasing to the esthetic sense, the ugly will be disagreeable in appearance and displeasing to the esthetic sense; and whereas the beautiful is constituted by order, proportion, symmetry, and harmony, the ugly results from disorder, disproportion, irregularity, and discord. The defects and blemishes which mar and disfigure objects and render them repulsive are either physical, intellectual, or moral. In fact, there are as many kinds and degrees of ugliness as there are of beauty. However, there is a neutral field between the beautiful and the ugly, the unbeautiful made up of things that are neither beautiful nor ugly, but occupy a place between the two. The beautiful, by slow and imperceptible degrees, shades off into the unbeautiful, and the unbeautiful as gradually merges into the positively ugly. As stated before (p. 62 sq.), it is impossible exactly to fix the

[1] Metaphysics Lect. 46, p. 628.

boundary lines between these regions; there can, however, be no doubt that these regions actually exist. — But as we are treating of ugliness only incidentally, these few remarks will suffice on this side issue.

# CHAPTER SIXTH

## BEAUTY IN RELATION TO GOD

### ARTICLE 1

#### DIVINE IDEALS THE MEASURE OF CREATED BEAUTY

Summary: Transition to new subject — Thesis — Proof of thesis.

73. **Transition to New Subject.** Hitherto we have viewed beauty in itself and in relation to the human faculties; in the next thesis we shall consider it in relation to God.

### THESIS 10

**The closer a beautiful object approaches its Divine ideal, the more beautiful it is.**

74. **Proof of Thesis.** To understand this statement we must first define what is meant by an ideal. An ideal is generally understood to be a conception regarded as a standard of perfection, that is, a conception free from all deformi-

ties, defects, or blemishes seen in actual existence. Now everything created or creatable has such an ideal of itself in the Divine mind. For God is the all-perfect Architect of the universe, the Artist of artists. But an artist always acts according to a preconceived model, and the more perfect the artist, the more perfect the model; hence God being the most excellent artist is guided in His work by models that fully express the perfection which a certain being can and should possess; and these models or standards are the Divine ideals of created or creatable things. Therefore the nearer a beautiful object comes to its ideal in the Divine mind, the more beautiful it is. As a matter of fact, created objects, especially if they are of a somewhat complex nature, very rarely reach the perfection of their models or ideals. Where is there a man, for instance, who has not his defects, and where is there an object in nature or art which does not fall short of perfection? This thought is well stated by Lessius: "Omnia possibilia continentur . . . in (divina) sapientia in exemplari formali in quo etiam existunt objective modo perfectissimo et illustrissimo; magis enim ibi fulgent quam in suis naturis creatis."[1] In the vernacular, "All possible things are contained in the (Divine) Intellect as in a true pattern in which they have objective existence in a most perfect

---

[1] De Perfectionibus Moribusque Divinis, l. 5, c. 2, 19.

and excellent manner; for there they shine forth with even greater luster than in their own created natures." Something similar is found in Longfellow's "Masque of Pandora" where he says:

> ... "The ideal beauty
> Which the creative faculty of mind
> Fashions and follows in a thousand shapes
> More lovely than the real."

## ARTICLE 2

### CREATED BEAUTY A REFLECTION OF UN-CREATED BEAUTY

**Summary:** Question stated — Thesis — Elucidation of thesis — Objection answered.

**75. Question Stated.** In the last article we considered created beauty in respect to the Divine ideals. It remains for us to show in what precise relation it stands to the Divine essence.

## THESIS 11

**All created beauty is but a faint reflection of the beauty of the Divine essence.**

**76. Elucidation of Thesis.** This assertion is merely an inference of the broader truth that all things whatever, whether actual or possible, are contained in the Godhead, not, indeed, just as they are in themselves with all their defects and limitations, but in an infinitely higher manner, in an " eminent " manner, to use a technical expression.

That all things are in some manner contained in God's essence is plain. For, were it not so, there would be some perfection outside of God, that is in no way in Him; but this is opposed to God's infinity, which is the boundless ocean of *all* reality. That finite things are in the Godhead in an infinitely higher degree than they are in themselves, likewise follows from God's infinity, since whatever is in God, is God and is consequently infinitely perfect. God then is the superlatively excellent Exemplar of all finite beings; finite beings, on the other hand, are copies of God, but falling infinitely short of Him in perfection; they are, as it were, the footprints of the Creator in the sands of time, His image dimly traced in His handiworks. Hence we infer that created beauty is a faint reflection of the beauty of God, who is not only beautiful, but Beauty itself, the "splendor veri " and the " splendor ordinis " in the very highest sense of the word. He is unlimited in the variety of His perfections, and yet possessed of the greatest conceivable unity, since in Him perfections infinite in number and degree are all identified with His essence. — To confirm what

we have said by a passage from St. Thomas [1]:
" Pulchritudo enim creaturæ nihil aliud est quam
similitudo divinæ pulchritudinis in rebus partici-
pata," that is, " The beauty of the creature is
nothing else than Divine beauty shared by
things."

77. **Objection Answered.** But, it is urged,
how can God be beautiful in the *true* sense of the
word, since beauty is order, and order in God is
inconceivable? For order requires divers parts,
and parts in God have no place.

This objection need not disturb us. For to
have order, it is not necessary to have parts
actually separable or even really distinct; it is
enough to have parts in the sense that one and
the same object be equivalent to many perfections
which are in harmony with one another. Now
this is the case with God. For, as reason teaches
us, the Divine essence, though excluding everything in the nature of parts, is nevertheless
equivalent to endless perfections which stand in
the most orderly relation to one another. — We
refrain from speaking of the great mystery of
the Ever Blessed Trinity, of Three in One, as
this is known to us by revelation only.

[1] In expositione in Dionys. c. 4, I. 5.

# CHAPTER SEVEN

## Objectivity of Beauty

**Summary:** Transition to new subject — Thesis — Exact scope of thesis explained — Thesis established.

**78. Transition to New Subject.** We now pass to the examination of a question which really follows as a corollary from what precedes, but which, on account of its importance and the opposition it has met with, needs more detailed treatment, namely the objectivity of beauty.

## THESIS 12

Beauty is not subjective, but objective.

**79. Exact Scope of Thesis.** It is not our purpose in this thesis to disprove the doctrine of idealism according to which *all* reality, and hence also beauty, is in its nature psychical, i.e. existent only in the mind. For this system is so utterly opposed to common sense as to deserve no consideration here. It is our intention rather to weigh the merits of the view according to which beauty consists essentially in certain *mental* qualities capable of being stimulated into action by outer objects. These outer objects, however, it is held, are not in themselves beautiful; they are merely excitants of delightful emotions and outward signs of the beauty within the soul. Hence this theory makes beauty wholly subjective. But it will be well to let one of the advocates of this theory, David Hume, speak for himself. He says in his dissertation " Of the Standard of Taste ": " Though it be certain that Beauty and Deformity, more than sweet and bitter, are not qualities in objects, but belong entirely to sentiment, it must be allowed that there are certain qualities in objects which are fitted by nature to produce particular feelings."

Now what is to be thought of this view? We answer, it is opposed to well-established conclusions, it leads to scepticism, and it, moreover, rests on confusion of ideas.

**80. Thesis Established.** And first, the view that beauty is subjective is opposed to well-established conclusions. In a previous thesis we showed that beauty consists in symmetry, harmony, proportion; briefly, in order. But order is something objective. For it results from the relations existing between the elements constituting a thing. Now if the elements constituting a thing are objective — and who will deny this but a confirmed sceptic? — the relations obtaining between these elements will also be objective. You might just as well say that the angles and the sides of a triangle are real, but that the relations between them are purely subjective.

Again, the view we are refuting leads to scepticism. For if the concept of beauty is not objective, what right have we to ascribe objectivity to any other concept, as substance, cause, virtue, goodness? They are all on a par with beauty as far as objectivity is concerned. They are all regarded as objective because the mind clearly represents them as objective. And if we are deceived by the mind as to the objectivity of beauty, are we not justified in deducing that the same is the case in regard to all other concepts?

Lastly, the opinion that beauty is purely subjective rests on a confusion of ideas. For it confounds the susceptibility to beauty with beauty itself, it mistakes the effect for the cause. We do not deny that the mind is so constituted as to be filled with delight when certain objects are presented to it. However, this constitution of the intellect thus to react at the sight of those objects is not beauty itself, but a disposition, a prerequisite for the enjoyment of beauty. Nor do we question that the joy of the mind consequent upon the perception of the beautiful is subjective, but this joy is not beauty itself, it is merely the effect of beauty.

We might also inquire of the upholders of the

view under discussion why it is that only *certain* objects excite those sentiments in which beauty is supposed to consist. If beauty is nothing in the object why should one object have the advantage over another in arousing the sense of beauty?

# CHAPTER EIGHT

## THE STANDARD OF TASTE

**Summary:** Connection with previous thesis pointed out — Thesis — Proof of thesis — Confirmation of thesis — Saying, "there is no disputing about tastes," explained — Diversity of tastes often only apparent — Corollary: Beauty not a transcendental concept.

**81. Connection with Previous Thesis Pointed out.** The thesis establishing the objectivity of beauty enables us to give a satisfactory answer to the much debated question as to whether there exists a fixed standard of taste.

## THESIS 13

**There exists a fixed standard of taste, and hence taste is not arbitrary.**

**82. Proof of Thesis.** Taste, as here understood, is the power of discerning and estimating the beautiful.[1] That there is a fixed standard of taste follows as a corollary from the preceding thesis. For if beauty is objective the concept of beauty is also objective, and therefore fixed,

[1] Cf. Liberatore, Log. et Metaph. p. 302.

definite, and determinate. Now the concept of beauty is the standard of taste, namely that by which we estimate or pass judgment on what is beautiful. Consequently, the standard of taste is likewise fixed, definite, and determinate, and hence taste is not dependent on each one's individual disposition, is not subject to each individual's caprice and private judgment, but is governed by fixed rule and law, in a word, it is not arbitrary.

83. **Confirmation of Thesis.** What we have thus shown by an a priori argument is confirmed by an appeal to common sense. For if there is no common standard of taste, if taste varies according to every individual's personal disposition, why is it that painters, sculptors, poets, architects, and other artists think that the fame of their works will be eternal and that their productions will please to the end of time? Such was the opinion of Horace who tells us:

"Exegi monumentum aere perennius,
  Regalique situ pyramidum altius;
  Quod non imber edax, non aquilo impotens
  Possit diruere, aut innumerabilis
  Annorum series, et fuga temporum.
  Non omnis moriar; multaque pars mei
  Vitabit Libitinam . . ."[1]

These lines have been thus rendered by Lord Lytton:

[1] Ode 3, 30.

"I have built a monument than bronze more lasting,
Soaring more high than regal pyramids,
Which nor the stealthy gnawing of the rain-drop,
Nor the vain rush of Boreas shall destroy;
Nor shall it pass away with the unnumbered
Series of ages and the flight of time.
I shall not wholly die! From Libitina
A part, yea, much of mine own self escapes."

As a matter of fact, the masterpieces of antiquity, as the poems of Homer, Virgil, Horace, Shakespeare, the statues of Michael Angelo, the paintings of Raphael, the architectural works of the Middle Ages, give as much delight now as they did when first produced.

Again, why is it that numerous books have been written laying down rules and directions which every artist must observe under penalty of producing a fiasco?

Lastly, why do we say that certain productions are in good or in bad taste? Such an expression has no meaning unless there is a fixed standard of taste to which the productions in question conform or from which they depart. If taste were altogether arbitrary, then whatever pleased the fancy of the individual beholder would be beautiful, and we would have no right to quarrel with a man for his tastes. If he judged the Moses of Michael Angelo ugly and the drama of "Hamlet" abominable we could not justly censure his taste.

**84. Saying "There is no Disputing about**

tastes," **Explained.** But what about the saying " De gustibus non est disputandum," " There is no debating about tastes " ? Does not the diversity of tastes among men as expressed in this generally accepted axiom prove that there is no common standard of taste? No, it no more shows this than the many errors and sins into which men are constantly falling show that there is no common standard of truth or morality. The axiom merely states the fact that there are many departures from good taste owing to personal peculiarities, uncommon surroundings, and other accidental or exceptional conditions and circumstances. To realize this, observe that there is a twofold element in taste, a perceptional and an emotional. As regards the perceptional element, taste imports discernment or the power of nice and correct judgment as to what is beautiful. Now the power of discerning what is beautiful is not ordinarily possessed in a very high degree of perfection; for, as stated before (p. 70), nature is not lavish of those gifts the purpose of which is adornment and enjoyment rather than necessity. Thus a talent for music is comparatively rare, because music is an endowment bestowed chiefly for enjoyment. The case is similar in regard to taste for beauty. No wonder, then, that so many blunders are committed in determining what is beautiful. Hence the diversity of judgment in respect to what is beautiful is not due to the fact that there is no common standard of taste, but to the fact that many possess little or no taste.

At times the taste is perverted in one who has associated with others that have no proper appreciation of the beautiful. Thus it may come about that a false standard of taste is gradually set up for an entire country and the taste of the inhabitants permanently vitiated. The perversion of taste in this instance is evidently the result of peculiar surroundings and accidental circumstances.

The emotional element of taste consists in the power of relishing or enjoying the beautiful. Now it is well known that the emotional capacities of men are very various. Some persons are more impressionable than others and hence more easily moved by beauty. Overlooking this fact, many ascribe to the outward cause alone the different estimates of beauty. These estimates are the joint effect of the object and the subject perceiving.

**85. Diversity of Tastes often only Apparent.** However, let it be noted by way of warning, the diversity of judgments in regard to the beauty of the same object is frequently only apparent, and this chiefly for two reasons. In the first place, sensible beauty, as explained thes. 7, p. 74 sqq., often consists in the realization by the mind of the proper adjustment between sense and object. Now it may happen, and frequently does happen, that what is in harmony with the sense-perception of one man is out of harmony with that of another, or, at any rate, less in harmony with it. Hence it is, for instance, that an Indian, considered handsome by one of his own tribe, is unattractive in the eyes of a white man. There is really no diversity in the estimation of beauty in this case. Both the Indian and the white man judge that adjustment and harmony are beautiful. The diversity of judgments is merely due to the fact that what is in keeping with the sense of the one, is out of keeping with the sense of the other. The Indian declares that to be beautiful which harmonizes with his sense of sight, and so does the white man. The white man is not aware of the reason why the Indian calls his fellow-tribesman handsome; hence he imagines that the Indian has a standard of beauty different from his own. Nor does this make beauty subjective; for the relation existing between sense and object is as objective as the object itself. Beauty would be subjective if it were made to consist merely in the subjective feeling, and not in the adjustment between the sensitive faculty and the object causing that feeling in the sensitive faculty. (Cf. p. 75.)

There is still a second reason why many judgments regarding the same object seem to be divergent, but in reality are not. It is this. An object is often beautiful considered from one standpoint and ugly considered from another. Two judgments disagree merely because they do not relate to the same object under the same *aspect*. Thus a boy calls a toad horrid because it displeases his sight; the scientist pronounces it beautiful on account of the perfect adjustment of all the parts of its organism. One is repelled by a person afflicted with a loathsome disease by reason of his appearance, another is attracted to him on account of his heroic patience. This is especially the case when the beauty of an object is due to association. You find your old homestead very beautiful. For the memory of the days of your boyhood spent in it casts a halo around it. Another, a stranger, thinks the same place very ordinary. And so in many other cases where perhaps the cause for the difference in judgments is not so evident. Were we to consider all these influences, we would understand that two persons who seem to be at variance in their estimates of beauty are really in full accord.

86. **Corollary: Beauty not a Transcendental Concept.** After treating the various questions regarding beauty, an answer can now be given to an enquiry often made. Is beauty like goodness a transcendental concept, a concept applicable to all things, in other words, can all things be called beautiful as all things can be called good?

If this question is taken in the strict sense, the reply is, no. For, as pointed out (thes. 5), things are not termed beautiful unless they are perfect in their own kind and unless they moreover possess a somewhat conspicuous degree of perfection. Now no one will contend that these two conditions are verified in everything. The case is different as regards the good; for a thing is called good by the very fact that it is something, that it is a reality. (See p. 22 sq.) However, in an improper sense, all things may be called beautiful in two ways. First they may be styled beautiful in so far as they can enter as parts into the constitution of beautiful things. A skeleton, although considered hideous, forms an essential part of every beautiful sentient being. Piles of stone, of lumber, and of cement have little or no beauty. But when combined so as to constitute, say the castle of Edinburgh, they are truly a thing of beauty. Hence it is correct to say that all things possess *potential* or *initial* beauty in so far as they can enter in some way or other into the constitution of beautiful things.— In the second place, anything may have symbolic beauty in the sense that it can be the token of something beautiful, as a wrinkled, emaciated face can be the token of a life well spent. Symbolic beauty, however, is not intrinsic beauty, but extrinsic beauty, it merely directs attention to something that is beautiful in itself.

# CHAPTER NINE

## VARIOUS FALSE SYSTEMS OF BEAUTY

**Summary:** Purpose of chapter set forth — Beauty and utility — Beauty and sensitive gratification —Beauty and the associationist theory — Beauty and custom — Pantheistic conception of beauty.

**87. Purpose of Chapter Set Forth.** Now that we have established the positive part of our treatise it remains for us to say something about the false theories of beauty, of which there are a considerable number. The chief of these theories are those which make beauty consist in utility, in pleasure of sense, in association, in custom, and in the Divine idea. They have been all refuted by implication before. For if our view of the beautiful is correct, then all other views at variance with it must be false. Nevertheless it will be useful to add a few words in direct refutation of them. However, our main purpose is not so much to refute these false theories as to point out how it came about that in this matter of beauty there exists such a multiplicity of views. The general reason for this great variety of views would seem to be the great

118

difficulty there is in disentangling beauty from its mere accompaniments, effects, and prerequisite conditions. In consequence of this difficulty, the mind is apt to confound beauty with one or other of those things which always or usually accompany it. Let us now show this in the case of each of the above opinions in particular.

**88. Beauty and Utility.** And first, as regards utility. That utility or usefulness constitutes beauty has been held by many. Socrates is credited with this view by Xenophon who in his "Memorabilia" 3, 8, makes him say: "Whatever is beautiful is for the same reason good, when *suited to the purpose* for which it was intended." And again, "Whatever is *suited for the end* intended, with respect to that end is good and fair; and contrariwise, it must be deemed evil and deformed when it departs from the purpose which it was designed to promote." He goes on to apply this theory of fitness to such things as houses. Those houses are most beautiful which are most convenient.[1] In modern times, similar views have been advanced by Adam Smith in "The Theory of Moral Sentiments," by Berkeley in "Alciphron," and by others.

As to this theory, it must be admitted that the useful is very frequently beautiful, not, however, just because it is useful, but because it shows

[1] See W. Knight, "The Philosophy of the Beautiful," v. I, p. 22.

forth fitness, proportion, adaptation of means to
end, in a word, because it involves order.   However, it does not follow that what is beautiful is
necessarily useful.   There are many things which
impress us as beautiful without any regard to
their usefulness, as the evening star rising above
the horizon, the foaming surge, a lion crouching
in the jungle, a hawk soaring on high.   But
when an object of a somewhat complex nature,
as a well constructed machine, is useful it is also
beautiful.   Nevertheless, although the useful and
the beautiful are often identified in external nature, they always differ in concept.   A thing is
considered useful in as far as it is helpful and
beneficial, and beautiful in as far as it stands in
*harmonious relation* to the end which it sub-
serves.   The reason then for confounding the
useful with the beautiful is the close connection
of the useful with the beautiful.

89. **Beauty and Sensitive Gratification.**
According to another view beauty relates only
to *sense* cognition and feeling.   The chief representative of this view is Alexander G. Baumgarten, the founder of the science of esthetics.
He says:  " Aesthetices finis est perfectio cog-
nitionis sensitivæ qua talis.   Hæc autem est pulchritudo," [1] " The end of esthetics is the perfection of sensuous cognition as such; and this is
beauty."  George T. Meier, Baumgarten's pupil,

---

[1] Aesthetica, 14.

following in the footsteps of his master, declares that "every perfection perceived by the senses is a *beauty,* and every sensible imperfection in like manner an ugliness." And for illustration he adds: "Wine tastes beautifully and flowers smell beautifully; music sounds beautifully and a handsome face looks beautifully." [1]

As regards this theory, we have shown in thesis 2 that the beautiful as such cannot be perceived by sense, but by the intellect only. No doubt, the apprehension of the beautiful is frequently accompanied by sensitive gratification of the eye and ear, both because charming sights and sounds are in harmony with the eye and ear and because intellectual delights often react on, and overflow into, the channels through which beautiful sensitive objects are transmitted to the mind. But beauty is one thing, and a mere accompaniment of beauty, quite another. Those philosophers, then, who mistake sensuous cognition and pleasure for beauty confound a mere concomitant of beauty with beauty itself, and thus degrade the enjoyment of the beautiful, one of the intellect's noblest prerogatives, to the low level of mere sensuous pleasure.

90. **Beauty and the Associationist Theory.** We now pass to the third false theory of the beautiful. This theory, which is quite common with English writers, makes beauty consist in

[1] Cf. Ueberweg, History of Philosophy, v. II, p. 117.

association. According to this view an object is beautiful because it is associated with, or suggests things which are calculated to arouse pleasurable feelings in us. Thus you find a nosegay sent you by a kind friend beautiful, because the thought of your friend's love and fidelity, which the present suggests, gives rise to agreeable emotions in you. — An old, faded copy-book is beautiful in your eyes, because it stirs up in you sweet recollections of the days of your youth and of your efforts and struggles and final success. But lest we may seem to be beating the air by refuting imaginary enemies, let us set down the statements of two representatives of this view, Mr. Alison and Lord Jeffrey. Mr. Alison says: "The conclusion in which I wish to rest is that the beauty and sublimity which is felt in the various appearances of matter are finally to be ascribed to their expression of mind, or to their being either directly or indirectly the *signs* of these qualities of mind which are fitted by the constitution of our nature to affect us with pleasing and interesting emotion."[1] And Lord Jeffrey formulates his view thus: "It appears to us, then, that objects are sublime or beautiful — first, when they are the natural *signs* and perpetual *concomitants* of pleasurable sensations, as the sound of thunder, or laughter, or at any rate, of some lively feeling or emotion in ourselves, or

[1] Essay on the Nature and Principles of Taste.

in some other sentient beings; or secondly, when they are the arbitrary or accidental concomitants of such feelings, as ideas of female beauty; or thirdly, when they bear some analogy or fancied resemblance to things with which these emotions are necessarily connected. All poetry is founded on the last — as silence and tranquillity — gradual decay and ambition — gradual descent and decay." [1] To make the meaning of the associationists still clearer we shall cite another passage from Lord Jeffrey's "Essay on Beauty." "Our sense of beauty," he says, " depends entirely on our previous experience of simpler pleasures or emotions and consists in the *suggestion* of agreeable and interesting sensations with which we had formerly been made familiar, by the direct agency of our common sensibilities; and that vast variety of objects to which we give the common name of beautiful become entitled to that appellation *merely* because they all possess the power of recalling or reflecting those sensations of which they have been the accompaniments, or with which they have been associated in our imagination by any other more casual bond of connection."

Now what is to be said of the theory of the associationists? If the theory merely maintains that there is a kind of beauty generally called symbolic, it is perfectly sound; but if it upholds,

[1] Article "Beauty" in the Encyclopædia Britannica.

as it actually does, that all beauty whatever consists in association, then it is full of inconsist-
encies. For if a thing is beautiful because it
suggests a pleasing emotion we naturally ask, Is
the emotion which is suggested beautiful or is it
not? If it is, we wish to know why. Is it because the pleasing emotion suggests another
pleasing emotion or is it because the pleasing
emotion is beautiful in itself? If the emotion is
beautiful because it suggests another agreeable
emotion, this second emotion will, in its turn, be
beautiful because it suggests a third agreeable emotion and so on forever. Hence in this supposition beauty would be without a foundation, without an ultimate support, without anything to give
it its beauty, and consequently no beauty at all.
— But if our opponents say that the emotion suggested is *in itself* beautiful, then they evidently
abandon their contention that *all* beauty results
from association.

Next let us see what would follow if the
associationists should take the other horn of
the original dilemma and say that the emotion
suggested possesses no beauty in itself. If this
be the case, namely if the emotion suggested
by an object is not beautiful, neither can it
impart beauty to the object suggesting it. For
nothing can impart to another what it does not
itself possess. We see then that the doctrine
making *all* beauty consist in association leads to

many contradictions and consequently is an illogical doctrine. This conclusion is confirmed by William Knight: " Jeffrey's theory is an irrelevancy from first to last, even more than Alison's." [1] The mistake of the associationists arises from the confusion of symbolical (extrinsic) beauty with beauty in general. Seeing that some things are beautiful owing to association, they infer that all beauty results from association.

91. **Beauty and Custom.** Another view somewhat akin to the one just rejected identifies beauty with custom, fashion, and habit. One of the representatives of this view is Sir Joshua Reynolds who in a discourse delivered to the students of the Royal Academy says: " We admire beauty for no other reason than that we are used to it. I have no doubt that if we were more used to deformity than beauty, deformity would then lose the idea annexed to it and take that of beauty, and that, if the whole world would agree that *yes* and *no* should change their meaning, *yes* would then deny and *no* would affirm."— According to this view then an object or a practice is beautiful, because we have grown familiar with it, whether this familiarity rests on a custom of the nation or community to which we belong, or on a prevailing fashion, or on a personal habit acquired through a frequent repetition of the same

act. For a better understanding of this theory
consider a few instances: The people of one
country regard a certain style of building, a certain cut of dress, certain fashions of social intercourse as most appropriate and beautiful, whereas
the people of another country consider the same
style, cut, and fashions as most odd, singular,
and laughable. In some parts of the Orient, a
man without a beard is looked upon with dis-
favor, in the West, a beardless man may be regarded as handsome. The inhabitants of some
regions imagine that they are attractively dressed
when their clothes display all the colors of the
rainbow, but the people of other countries are of
an altogether opposite opinion. Custom would
seem to be the only way to account for this diversity of tastes.— In ancient times, gladiatorial
shows were held in Rome. Men fought with
each other or with wild beasts in the arena before
immense crowds of spectators. These contests
were thought to be splendid exhibitions of human prowess and worthy to be attended by the
flower of the nation. We, in our day, turn from
such scenes of carnage with horror and loathing.
No excuse can be urged for such practices except that they were the custom in those days.—
To add another example from the domain of language where custom seems to reign supreme.
That pronunciation and accentuation of words
appear beautiful to you to which you have been

accustomed. If you leave your home and settle down among people who pronounce and accentuate differently from the way to which you are used, you feel at first disgusted at the novel mode of oral expression. But gradually the peculiarities of language in the new locality lose their strangeness and grow agreeable. Custom makes all the difference.— These are facts. Do they prove that custom constitutes beauty, do they show that a thing is beautiful because we are accustomed to it, and ugly because we are not accustomed to it? No, they do not. They prove only that custom is *often* closely associated with beauty, but not that custom is beauty. Custom and habit cannot be beauty; for beauty is in the thing, it is objective; habit and custom are in the one contemplating beauty, they are subjective.— Again, many things strike us as beautiful on first acquaintance. In fact, first impressions are often the strongest, so much so that some philosophers, going to the other extreme, have identified beauty with novelty. When you saw the rainbow for the first time you found it beautiful, perhaps more than ever after. When you heard the organ peal forth its rich, full notes on your first visit to church you were charmed, may be, more intensely than at any other time.— Lastly, there are many things to which no acquaintance, no matter how long, can reconcile us. A sightless man never appears beautiful, even though we see him ever so often. An ungrateful child will always be an abomination in our sight.

However, there exists a very intimate connection between custom and beauty, and it is on account of this connection that beauty has been confounded with custom. This connection we shall now endeavor to trace.— Long, familiar acquaintance with an object, in the first place, gives us an opportunity of finding out its good points. Hence custom, though not beauty, may be an indispensable condition for the realization of beauty; for it helps to promote clearness of perception, which we showed to be a necessary prerequisite for the due perception of beauty (thesis 6). How often has it not happened that two destined to be bosom-friends, on first meeting, looked at each other askance and mistrusted one another? It was only gradually, after long fellowship, that the beautiful qualities of each broke upon the other and that the links of friendship which nothing could sever, were forged.— People of different nationalities would not dislike one another as they sometimes do, if the barriers of diversity of language, rendering mutual intercourse and exchange of ideas difficult, were removed.

A second reason why custom makes attractive what at first repelled is this. By living in certain conditions and surroundings habitually, our physical and mental attitude towards certain things changes and thus what once offended us, now pleases. The object itself has not become beautiful through custom or habit, but *we* have changed under the long continued influence of our new conditions and surroundings, and consequently we now stand in different relation to the object. It is in this matter of beauty pretty much as it is with organic tastes. Here is some one who has left his home and taken up his abode with strangers. Many of their dishes in the beginning repelled him; but little by little his system adapted itself to their diet, and now he partakes of their food with as much relish as any of the rest. Think of the nausea and misery the first cigar caused that inveterate smoker. Habit has made delightful what in the beginning was almost a torture. Custom acts in a similar manner in the case of beauty. A certain way of acting, a certain fashion of dress, a certain tune, the features of some man or the appearance of some animal at first fills us with aversion and repugnance. But little by little we adjust ourselves to these things; we are no longer out of harmony with them; consequently what seemed so offensive before, appears attractive now. Hence custom and habit are not beauty, but they often aid in establishing adjustment, agreement, harmony between the subject perceiving and the object perceived.

92. **Pantheistic Conception of Beauty.** There is still one more false system concerning

the nature of beauty which it will be useful to notice, namely the system which identifies beauty with the Divine idea, with God revealing Himself in the finite, with the Absolute realizing itself in the relative. The advocates of this view are chiefly Schelling and Hegel. Thus in the opinion of Schelling, "the infinite finitely represented is beauty. Where beauty is, there the infinite contradiction is removed in the object itself." [1] With Hegel "the beautiful is the absolute in sensuous existence, the actuality of the idea in the form of limited manifestation." [2]

These descriptions of beauty recall what we said of the relation of the beautiful to the Divine ideals of which the beautiful objects are copies (theses 10 and 11). However, it is hardly possible to connect the doctrines of such men as Schelling and Hegel with our own. For their doctrines are based on pantheistical and, therefore, radically false views of philosophy, namely on the assumption that God is the world, and consequently that there is no personal God. On this account, there is no point of contact between our doctrine on beauty and theirs.

[1] Cf. Ueberweg, History of Philosophy, v. II, p. 219.
[2] Ibid., p. 242.

# CONCLUSION

We have thus completed our treatise on the beautiful. We started out by directing attention to an effect which the beautiful produces, namely delight in the one contemplating it. We next inquired into the relations of the beautiful to our cognitive faculties and found that the senses as such are incapable of perceiving the beautiful and that, consequently, the intellect alone is capable of doing so. We then asked ourselves what kind of delight the beautiful engendered in the soul. We arrived at the conclusion that beauty as *such* produces none but intellectual delight and that it excites love in the soul only in so far as it is identified with the good. Having settled these preliminary questions we ascertained that the essence of beauty consists in the "splendor of order," and further that for beauty to be fully appreciated and enjoyed, it must be clearly perceived by the mind. We next passed on to the investigation of sensible beauty as a preparatory step to the investigation of the beauty most congenial to man, namely spiritual beauty manifested through an appropriate sensible symbol. From the consideration of beauty in itself we turned

131

to the consideration of beauty in relation to God, the pattern and source of all finite beauty. After this we showed that beauty is not a mere internal feeling, but something objective and that, consequently, there exists a fixed standard of taste. In the last chapter we enumerated the chief false systems of beauty and subjected them to a critical examination according to the principles laid down before.

Man lives then in a world of beauty, but this beauty is from above, from the infinite, uncreated Beauty of God, the All-Beautiful.

# ALPHABETICAL INDEX

# From Saint Pius X Press

| | |
|---|---|
| Bernadette of Lourdes | 25.00 |
| Characteristics of True Devotion | 12.00 |
| Conference Matter For Religious | 25.00 |
| Eternal Punishment | 15.00 |
| Holiness Of Life | 15.00 |
| Holy Week Manual For Servers | 15.00 |
| Mercy Is Forever | 16.00 |
| New Lights On Pastoral Problems | 15.00 |
| Peter's Name | 15.00 |
| Practical Method of Reading the Breviary | 20.00 |
| Readings For Each Sunday In The Year | 12.95 |
| Sanctity in America | 16.00 |
| Sister Faustina: Apostle of Divine Mercy | 15.00 |
| Spiritual Maxims | 18.00 |
| The Art of Prayer | 20.00 |
| The Christian Trumpet | 25.00 |
| The Cult of Our Lady | 15.00 |
| The Divine Office | 15.00 |
| The Mirror of the Blessed Virgin Mary and The Psalter of Our Lady | 25.00 |
| The Possibility of Invincible Ignorance of the Natural Law | 30.00 |
| The Precepts of the Church | 15.00 |
| The Present Crisis of the Holy See | 15.00 |
| The Religious State | 11.95 |
| The True Story of the Vatican Council | 20.00 |
| The Virtues Of A Religious Superior | 15.00 |
| Vocations | 9.95 |

Saint Pius X Press

Box 74
Delia KS 66418
www.stpiusxpress.com

If you have a book that you are looking for to be reprinted and we do not have it listed, contact us at contact@stpiusxpress.com